THE REALITY OF RECOVERY IN PERSONALITY DISORDER

by the same author

Personality Disorder
Temperament or Trauma?
Heather Castillo
ISBN 978 1 84310 053 9
eISBN 978 1 84642 377 2

of related interest

Personality Disorder
The Definitive Reader
Edited by Gwen Adshead and Caroline Jacob
ISBN 978 1 84310 640 1
eISBN 978 1 84642 864 7
Forensic Focus Series

The Pits and the Pendulum
A Life with Bipolar Disorder
Brian Adams
ISBN 978 1 84310 104 8
eISBN 978 1 84642 358 1

Family Experiences of Bipolar Disorder
The Ups, The Downs and the Bits In Between
Cara Aiken
ISBN 978 1 84310 935 8
eISBN 978 0 85700 387 4

THE REALITY OF RECOVERY IN PERSONALITY DISORDER

HEATHER CASTILLO

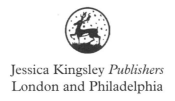

Jessica Kingsley *Publishers*
London and Philadelphia

The excerpt on page 203 from *The Fellowship of the Ring* by J.R.R. Tolkien is reprinted by permission of HarperCollins Publishers Ltd © The Tolkien Estate Limited 1954, 1955, 1966.

First published in 2016
by Jessica Kingsley Publishers
73 Collier Street
London N1 9BE, UK
and
400 Market Street, Suite 400
Philadelphia, PA 19106, USA

www.jkp.com

Library of Congress Cataloging in Publication Data
Castillo, Heather, author.
  The reality of recovery in personality disorder / Heather Castillo.
    p. ; cm.
  Includes bibliographical references and index.
  ISBN 978-1-84905-605-2 (alk. paper)
  I. Title.
  [DNLM: 1. Haven Project. 2. Community Mental Health Services--Great Britain. 3. Personality
Disorders--therapy--Great Britain. 4. Evidence-Based Medicine--Great Britain. WM 190]
  RC473.P56
  616.85'81--dc23
                            2015005796

British Library Cataloguing in Publication Data
A CIP catalogue record for this book is available from the British Library

ISBN 978 1 84905 605 2
eISBN 978 1 78450 071 9

Printed and bound in Great Britain

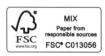

Dedicated to the dear old Haven

Contents

Acknowledgements

This book represents a journey which is a highly significant part of my life and the many people who have journeyed with me are, therefore, very dear to my heart.

First, I would like to thank Professor Shula Ramon, who has guided me through two research endeavors and who has been my touchstone and my great inspiration for collaborative research with service users. Thank you, also, to Dr Nicola Morant, whose dogged adherence to sound research methodology was often resented at the time, truthfully, but deeply appreciated in retrospect.

I would like to thank my publishers, especially Jessica Kingsley herself, for believing in this book. Also my husband, Alex, who has put up with quite a lot and who has continued to listen to, and read, so many drafts of what I have written, for so many years, with mostly forbearance and a few moans here and there, it has to be said. Thank you for believing in me, in all of us, and in what we aimed to achieve. Couldn't have done it without you.

Thank you to those in the National Personality Disorder team for their trust and support, Nick Benefield, Dr Rex Haigh, Frankie, Sue and all, not forgetting Kath Lovell at Emergence. What a time of innovation and fruitfulness we had. Thanks are also due to Reg McKenna, Haven Chairman, and to The Haven Board of Directors for so much support during my time as Chief Executive and research initiator. Profound thanks to the wonderful Haven staff team for all the laughs (bunch of jokers) and for all their unbelievable hard work and dedication over the years.

To thank, individually, all of the service users I have worked with during this time would constitute pages of names. There is a sea of much-loved faces before me. Your courage, hopefulness, and humour have been amazing. What we accomplished was achieved by all of us. To those in the research group, and those who took part in the research events, your words are reflected again and again throughout the pages of this book. I will, however, mention a few of you by name. Thank you to Dee Graham, who committed to facilitating groups and interviews during our research with such love and care. Finally, thank you to dear Becky and Helen. Helen Price, the client lead at The Haven for so many years, and Becky Attwater, who was in it from the start. Both so dedicated and such enduring comrades on the journey.

CHAPTER 1

The Journey Begins

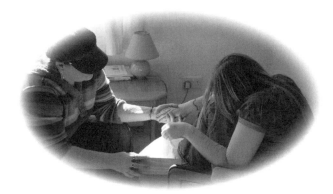

Nearly every other day I was tying things around my neck, overdosing, cutting myself, starving myself ... I used to wake up every day, wanting to die, finding a way, thinking of a way that I could harm myself when I was in hospital, trying to trick people into like thinking I was okay, trying to sneak things in, but looking around constantly for something I could do, and that was my life, trying to find a way to actually harm myself. I didn't want to live. I didn't have any hopes or dreams. I just thought my life was going to be in hospital.

Service User Quotation

This book tells of a journey taken by a group of service users who had attracted a diagnosis of personality disorder, a journey that spans 20 years. It is an account that aspires to show the inner world of personality disorder from the perspective of service users. It aims to examine the process of recovery for those with this diagnosis and it suggests evidence-based ways forward for support and treatment. It is both a cautionary tale and a story of hope.

Some lives appear to have fault lines running through them, fatal flaws. It was in the early 1990s, in North East Essex in England that I first stepped into a psychiatric ward. I saw a young woman with cuts covering her arms. I wondered who could have done such a thing to her, not realizing that they were self-inflicted. I did not know how or why such acts should come to be. I did not understand why human beings, who held a life in common with me, should be driven to such acts. Here was the beginning of my particular part of this journey.

At that time, as a mental health advocate working for Mind organizations in North East Essex, and based at the local psychiatric acute inpatient hospital, the advocacy office was a frequent port of call for service users with a diagnosis of personality disorder. The themes they brought were consistent: discharge from hospital immanent even though still suicidal; being sectioned into hospital under the Mental Health Act and subject to close observation; being transferred to a secure hospital; at risk of losing children via child protection procedures; ending in prison; and a whole gamut of desperate outcomes, all contributing to a compounding of symptoms and feelings of being fundamentally and irrevocably misunderstood.

One man wandered aimlessly into the Mind office saying that the psychiatrist had told him there was nothing that could be done for him because he had personality disorder. Later that year he was dead. A woman in the local psychiatric hospital ward, who was self-starving to a dangerous degree, was told in exasperated terms that she simply needed to start eating. These were not isolated examples and I became consumed with questions about this diagnosis. As an advocate I became the listener...to stories about lives where there seemed no mercy, where the world appeared treacherous and full of chaos and without reason and where the effects of time, visible and invisible, had dissolved hope. At that time I was involved in a kind of mental health advocacy that I believe has gone out of fashion. This was advocacy used to articulate the views of people generally not heard. It was advocacy inspired by such activists as Larry Gostin, the American lawyer who was the first legal director of National Mind, and whose book *A Human Condition* (1975) was largely responsible for reforms embraced in the UK 1983 Mental Health Act. I questioned whether, as an advocate, I could be the purveyor of stories of suffering and injustice that might lead to understanding and change.

Consequently, by 1998, I had embarked on what was to be the first of two research studies about personality disorder diagnosis. Together with local service users, I formed a research group comprised of people who had attracted the diagnosis with the aim of carrying out research about personality disorder from the service users' perspective. The group met monthly throughout 1999. Attendees were not survivors engaged in a retrospective study, but were service users in the midst of their difficulties, struggling for emotional equilibrium while engaged in the research endeavour. Some were inpatients and came to the group meetings from hospital wards each month, some came even though sectioned under the Mental Health Act. In a client group considered inconsistent, undependable and untreatable, the dedicated commitment from participants provided a contradictory picture; it was breath-taking.

Our research approach was emancipatory. Described by Freire (1970) as a method which challenges the validity of the privileged effectively analyzing the underprivileged, here the research tools would be given to the people (Ramon, Castillo and Morant 2001). By December 1999 the final interview was completed and, capturing the voice of the sample, the data collected from the group and the questionnaires yielded a vast quantity of perspectives including 15,000 service user words. In a climate that emphasized issues of risk and danger, and where personality disorder was considered untreatable in many quarters, part of the purpose in carrying out the first study was to engender some kind of compassion and understanding in relation to this diagnosis.

The study consisted of 50 participants, 20 men and 30 women, aged between 18 and 74 years. At a time when early abusive experiences were not so readily linked to present condition, the findings revealed that 88 per cent of the sample had experienced abuse. For 80 per cent this was childhood abuse, sexual, emotional, violent, and sometimes combinations of all three, constituting brutal life experiences. Twenty per cent made the discovery that they had the diagnosis indirectly, from records, reports or at social services meetings. Others appear to have been told about the diagnosis after many years; some were told by professionals only after they had asked. Seventy-two per cent of respondents considered they had received bad treatment because of the label. Confirming that the diagnosis is stigmatizing, they described their experiences of being treated as a *'service leper', 'let's give her a wide berth', 'you're ignored', 'hostility', 'not mental illness', 'brought on oneself', 'people seem to be scared of the diagnosis', 'it's saying troublemaker'*. What service users said during the interviews highlighted the sense of exclusion and hopelessness connected to finding out they had been given this diagnosis, and gave some sense of the impact this information might have on an individual labouring with the desperately hard task of living with the truth of an early abusive history.

Data analysis questioned the validity of the classification of personality disorder and the sub-categories within it. For those involved in our study, unresolved trauma had resulted in suicide attempts of such lethality that survival seemed miraculous. Anger and hatred had become dammed up behind a narrow response function. Where early life had been sexually or violently abusive, or simply consisted of an unloving and devastating non-response from care-givers, the blunt limitations of their experience had left some stripped of control and disempowered beyond comprehension.

From the year 2000 we began to present our findings at national conferences and we published a number of journal articles. Interest in our endeavour was heartening and liberating for the service users involved in the study and it was eventually published as a book, *Personality Disorder: Temperament or Trauma?* (Castillo 2003). At this time we did not know that our journey was simply beginning and that there was still so far to travel.

CHAPTER 2

Prevailing Knowledge
Relevant to the Journey

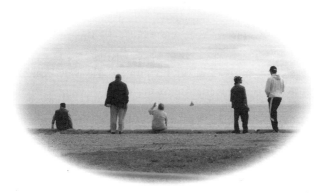

It is no wonder that those of us with a personality disorder diagnosis feel like second, or more like third class citizens (life's rejects). You only have to look at the definitions given in ICD 10 and DSM IV (the psychiatric diagnostic manuals) and read comments such as 'limited capacity to express feelings; disregard for social obligations; callous unconcern for others; deviant social behaviour; inconsiderate of others; incompetence; threatening or untrustworthy'. The list is endless, but one thing that these comments have in common is that they are not helpful in any way.

Service User Quotation

Before recounting the details of the next stage of our story, it is important to examine existing knowledge relevant to this journey. How does the law relate to personality disorder? What is personality disorder and what is its prevalence? What treatments have been developed and what is meant by recovery?

Mental health law

The Mental Health Act in the UK, relevant to England and Wales, covers the reception, care and treatment of mentally disordered people, the management of their property and other related matters. Centrally, it provides the legislation by which people diagnosed with a mental disorder can be detained in hospital or police custody, under a section of the Act, and can have their disorder assessed or treated against their wishes, colloquially known as 'sectioning'.

The term psychopathic disorder, used synonymously with personality disorder, became included in legislation in the 1959 Mental Health Act, with a clause in the 1983 Act requiring that those detained must be amenable to treatment to justify detention. Problems arose regarding the question of treatability and this remained a major consideration in proposed revisions of the 1983 Mental Health Act. Perhaps the most high profile event in relation to these concerns was the Russell murders (Edwards 2012). Michael Stone, a man diagnosed with personality disorder, had been discharged from psychiatric hospital as he was considered to be untreatable. In 1996, he went on to murder Dr Megan Russell and her six-year-old daughter while they were out walking their dog in a country meadow. Josie, the nine-year-old daughter who accompanied them, was attacked but survived. She was mute for some months and her appearance with her father on national television touched the nation's hearts. Brutal murder and personality disorder began to feature synonymously in the press. In July 1999, the Home Office issued policy proposals for managing dangerous people with severe personality disorder suggesting removal to special units, without deterioration in clinical state, if deemed potentially dangerous to the public (Department of Health 1999). This caused fairly widespread fear amongst those with the diagnosis, the vast majority of whom had harmed only themselves and not others. The advocacy service began to hear from anxious service users who had at some time received the diagnosis or who had at one time assaulted another, no matter how minor the offence. Notwithstanding assurances regarding the small number proposed for indeterminate detention, and their historical dangerousness, many were not calmed. Soon after, I heard a social worker speaking at a conference and likening the new proposals for preventative detention to the Tom Cruise film, *Minority Report.* Here a futuristic task force operates clairvoyant electronic equipment to predict the next time and place a crime will be committed and then identifies the culprit needing to be apprehended before they have actually perpetrated the crime. Many of us in the audience believed that this social worker who compared new Mental Health Act proposals to *Minority Report* had a point.

In December 1999, a unique coalition of 26 health organizations, disability, legal, civil rights and religious organizations published a joint statement expressing common concerns over government proposals for people diagnosed with severe personality disorder. Members of this coalition included The Church of England, The Community Psychiatric Nurses Association, The Law Society, The Mental Health Foundation, The Royal College of Psychiatrists, Community Health Councils, WISH (Women in Secure Hospitals), The United Kingdom Advocacy Network, National Mind and others. Issues highlighted included the exclusion from services of people with personality disorder; that there was no clear consensus regarding diagnosis; the difficulties inherent in risk assessment; the possibility of non-offenders (those who had not committed a criminal act) being detained against their will regardless of whether it was considered that they could be treated or not; the call for more research into what could best provide treatment and care for people with personality disorder, both those in the community and those detained in penal, restrictive establishments. This coalition became the Mental Health Alliance, a coalition of 75 organizations working together to secure better mental health legislation.

As illustrated above, the treatability clause in the 1983 Mental Health Act stipulated that someone so diagnosed, who presented a risk under the terms of the Act, could not be detained unless they were considered treatable. Proposals for an amended Act began with the replacement of the term *psychopathic disorder* with *personality disorder*. Continued concern was voiced nationally regarding the 'special attention' being accorded to the diagnosis of *personality disorder* and it was subsequently replaced by the term *mental disorder*. This single definition of mental disorder, as 'any disorder or disability of the mind', applies throughout the amended Act and abolishes references to categories of disorder. The 'treatability test' was replaced by an 'appropriate medical treatment test' characterized as meaning that medical treatment appropriate to that person's mental disorder is made available to them. In July 2007, after eight years of debate and controversy, the Mental Health Act 2007 was given Royal Assent and came into force the following year. Also, in July 2007, the Mental Health Alliance published its final report (Daw *et al.* 2007). In this report the Alliance concluded that some significant gains had been achieved by their campaign, citing one as the inclusion of medical treatment now being stipulated as something which alleviated or prevented worsening of the disorder, or one or more of its symptoms or manifestations. They suggested more work on the Code of Practice to ensure that this was appropriately interpreted.

Whether God or the devil is in the details, it is the details that suggest that 'small-print', or some logical thinking around the definitions above, might bring one to the conclusion that the fundamental detail here is, what is effective treatment? In the 1990s, as a mental health advocate, I was very concerned with the law and the Mental Health Act. Whilst continuing to acknowledge this as an important context, during the 2000s my attention turned to the issue of treatment.

The prevalence and impact of personality disorder

Coid *et al.* (2006) estimate that 4 per cent of people in Great Britain have a personality disorder. The British Psychological Society defines personality disorder as variations in or exaggerations of normal personality attributes, which are sometimes associated with anti-social behaviour (Alwin *et al.* 2006). Their report suggests that many people with mental health problems also have significant personality problems which reduce the effectiveness of their treatments. The British Psychological Society suggests that a higher proportion of the population than the Coid study above, 10 per cent, meet the criteria for a personality disorder diagnosis and that prevalence is much higher among psychiatric patients. The Personality Disorder Practitioner Guide (Department of Health 2014) advises that different research studies suggest between 5 and 12 per cent of the UK population would meet the criteria for a diagnosis of personality disorder. The Guide highlights its higher prevalence in relation to 1 per cent of the population who will have at least one episode of psychosis in their life and 2 per cent who suffer from major depression. The spectrum of difficulties for people diagnosed with personality disorder is also highlighted in the guide, ranging from relatively mild and needing treatment at times of stress to highly disabling.

The National Institute for Health and Clinical Excellence issued guidelines for the treatment and management of borderline personality disorder (NICE 2009). The Guidelines represent suicide attempts as a defining feature of the diagnosis with some studies suggesting that suicides can be as high as 10 per cent (Paris 2004). The economic impact of personality disorder has been highlighted with an estimated £704 million in health service costs per annum, predicted to rise to £1.1 billion by 2026 (McCrone *et al.* 2008).

What is personality disorder?

At the time of our initial study we noted that the American and European psychiatric diagnostic manuals referred to personality disorders as enduring patterns of behaviour that deviate markedly from the expectations of the individual's culture, and pervasive, inflexible deficits which are stable over time (DSM IV 1994; ICD 10 1992). This gave the service user little cause for any hope at all. It was a category about which considerable doubts had been expressed and it was a diagnosis which was often hidden from patients (Lewis and Appleby 1988).

In our first study we began our investigations with a history of the diagnosis of personality disorder. This history began over 200 years ago, when a French psychiatrist (Pinel 1801) spoke of *'manie sans delire'*, mania without delirium. Pritchard (1835, p.126) formulated the term 'moral insanity', which he defined as *'a morbid perversion of the natural feelings, affections, inclination, temper, habits, moral dispositions and natural impulses'*. Negative, judgemental and deeply moralistic language developed throughout the 19th century. Maudsley wrote, *'It is not our business, and it is not in our power, to explain psychologically the origins and nature of these depraved instincts, it is sufficient to establish their existence as facts of observation'* (Maudsley 1884, p.ix). Koch (1891) introduced the term psychopathic inferiority, and in 1905, Kraepelin was to replace 'inferiority' with 'personality'. He defined the psychopathic personality as falling into seven types, excitable, unstable, eccentric, liars, swindlers, anti-social and quarrelsome.

The Mental Deficiency Act (1913) added the term moral defective as a legislative control for detention of those considered to fall into this category. Schneider (1923) classified ten sub-categories of personality abnormalities of all types, ranging from those who caused suffering to others, to those causing suffering to themselves, including markedly depressive and insecure characters. By 1939, Henderson broadened classifications to include those prone to suicide, drug and alcohol abuse, pathological lying, hypochondria, instability and sensitivity. Borderline Personality Disorder was a concept which arose in the 1950s to describe people who were considered to be on the borderline between neurosis and

21

psychosis. This concept evolved into a personality disorder. It was classified in the Diagnostic and Statistical Manual of Mental Disorders, DSM I 1952, as sociopathic personality disturbance, and became included as borderline personality disorder in DSM III in 1980.

The first legal definition of psychopathy became contained within legislation, with criteria for detention, in the 1959 Mental Health Act. In the 1980s the term *severe personality disorder*, defined in relation to the severity of personality disturbance, began to be used (Kernberg 1984; Tyrer 1988). This term started to appear in government documents as *dangerous and severe personality disorder* (Department of Health 1999) and marked the beginning of action for revisions of the Mental Health Act. The concept of dangerous and severe personality disorder (DSPD) was considered to be a more extreme form of anti-social personality disorder, representing a dimension of serious risk to others.

At the time of completing our first study, the modern concept of personality disorder was captured in the ten sub-categories of the European diagnostic manual ICD 10 1992 and its transatlantic counterpart at that time, DSM IV 1994:

Paranoid personality disorder

Schizoid personality disorder

Schizotypal personality disorder

Anti-social or dissocial personality disorder

Borderline personality disorder or emotionally unstable impulsive type

Histrionic personality

Narcissistic personality disorder

Avoidant personality disorder

Dependent personality disorder

Obsessive-compulsive or anankastic personality disorder

Definitions of these categorizations are readily available in psychiatric texts. They outline a wide range of personality abnormalities, the clinical definitions range from the most timid, to the most dangerous among us. The diagnosis has contested scientific legitimacy and Pilgrim (2000) suggested that it is an elastic concept which may include a wide range of people and encompass a variety of presentations. DSM IV and ICD 10 definitions suggested that those with personality disorder may display certain behaviours or embody certain character traits; however, these definitions did not say why.

Although there are ten diagnostic sub-categories attributed to personality disorder, the two most commonly diagnosed are borderline personality disorder and dissocial/anti-social personality disorder. This was reflected in our research group, for the initial study, where all members had acquired either a borderline or dissocial diagnosis. Service users diagnosed with borderline personality disorder are characterized as emotionally unstable, impulsive and self-destructive, while dissocial personality disorder is described as a callous unconcern for others with deviant social behaviour and a potential for danger to one's fellows. Whether the categorization was borderline or dissocial, our earlier study showed high incidences of early abuse, self-harm and suicidality across both categories.

Psychiatric descriptions observe from the outside representing surface perceptions of feelings and behaviour. The experiences of service users in the first study revealed a profound subjectivity which described early events and feelings associated with dysfunctional behaviour. The sense of self was explored in terms of symptomatology including dissociative states and hearing voices. The quality of depression was expressed in relation to rejection, isolation and low self-esteem or unworthiness. Participants described their experiences in terms of self-blame and precipitants and their descriptions encompassed context rather than fixed behaviour. Some aspirations included compassion and the desire to change. The earlier study proposed a new construct about the disorder reformulated from the experiences and interpretations of those who had attracted a diagnosis of personality disorder. It highlighted an awareness of this classification as not so much a diagnosis, but as a poorly adapted coping mechanism.

In 2013, the fifth revision of the American diagnostic manual, *Diagnostic and Statistical Manual of Mental Disorders*, DSM 5, was published, 19 years after its predecessor, DSM IV. Earlier proposals tabled for DSM 5 would have significantly changed the method by which individuals are diagnosed. A growing awareness of the difficulties of fitting people into distinctly separate clinical syndromes, and the tendency for overlapping symptomatology, gave rise to suggestions that a dimensional approach to diagnosis should replace the current trait/categorical model for personality disorder. However, the American Psychiatric Association ultimately decided to retain the DSM IV categorical approach with the same ten personality

23

disorders. An alternative hybrid dimensional-categorical model has been featured in a separate chapter in Section III of DSM 5. The alternative model is included to encourage further study into how this new approach could be used to assess personality and diagnose personality disorders in clinical practice. Here the clinician would note the severity of impairment in personality functioning and the problematic personality trait(s). The hybrid approach retains six personality disorder types:

Borderline personality disorder

Obsessive-compulsive personality disorder

Avoidant personality disorder

Schizotypal personality disorder

Anti-social personality disorder

Narcissistic personality disorder

Meantime, former service user and recovery guru Ron Coleman, has, as a bit of serious fun, irreverently produced DSM Zero, 'Everything You Need to Know about Your Mental Health' (2014).

During our research study in the 1990s, our examination of the 200-year history of the diagnosis caused us to conclude that it was characterized by confusion and lack of agreement and, where understanding was required, fear had emerged. In the research report for our initial study (Castillo 2003) we inserted a table which illustrates the history we had uncovered and it is included here again (Table 2.1), as a graphic depiction of the early pejorative and inconsistent history of the diagnosis. The current addition at the end of the table illustrates little conceptual progress.

Table 2.1 Historical context

Date	Description	Author/text
1801	'Manie sans deleire' (mania without delirium)	Pinel
1835	Moral insanity	Pritchard
1857	Degenerative deviation (moral imbecility)	Morel
1876	The unborn criminal	Lombroso
1884	'No capacity for true moral feeling'	Maudsley
1891	Psychopathic inferiority	Koch
1905	Psychopathic personality	Kraepelin
1913	Moral defective – mental deficiency act	Mental Deficiency Act
1923	Psychopathy – 10 sub-classifications	Schneider
1939	Three groups of psychopaths	Henderson
1941	The mask of sanity	Cleckley
1950s	Borderline personality disorder	DSM I
1959	Psychopathic disorder	The Mental Health Act
1980s	Severe personality disorder	Kernberg, Tyrer
1990s	10 sub-classifications (traits)	DSM IV & ICD 10
1999	Dangerous severe personality disorder	DoH & Home Office
2013	10 sub-classifications (traits)	DSM 5

The next edition of the European Diagnostic Manual, ICD 11, is due to be published in 2017. In recognition of the fact that the impact of personality traits are variable in severity, proposals for ICD 11 are likely to include reference to severity of impairment in personality functioning.

The trait or categorical method of diagnosis describes surface manifestations and fails, fundamentally, to capture the experiences of the sufferer. Because of the current unreliability of the diagnosis, making it difficult to translate into practice, some already choose to see personality disorder as a unitary syndrome (Adshed and Jacob 2009). In order to capture what is individual and unique for someone, developing a *formulation* is suggested (Department of Health 2014). This attempts to describe the range of factors contributing to that person's difficulties and guides the support and development of management strategies.

The over-pathologizing of human behaviour is something that has been debated from Szasz (1961) to present-day responses to DSM 5 (Cooke and McGowan 2014). However, at the time of our original study we believed that resources were currently focused in the psychiatric area and we feared that, if personality disorder were to become demedicalized, too many people in need of support might become abandoned or criminalized. We dreamed of a better way where sufferings and their causes would be understood, where individuals would be seen as multi-dimensional and where their strengths would not go unacknowledged. Although it is true that contested validity might, to some degree, be applied to other psychiatric diagnoses, the trait classification of the medical model of personality disorder, in particular, still suggests that the condition can be negatively enduring.

26

The medical model and the concept of cure

The biomedical model of illness and health care understands concepts such as illness, remission and relapse. In psychiatry the conferring of a diagnosis has the potential to affect those concepts, instilling beliefs about the notion of cure. The psychiatric diagnostic manuals have suggested that, although most patients with schizophrenia will improve with treatment, relatively few recover to such an extent that they are back to normal. They refer to personality disorders as enduring patterns of behaviour and pervasive, inflexible deficits that are stable over time. Medical treatments have relied on intermittent hospitalization and the prescribing of medication.

For many with a personality disorder diagnosis, being treated in primary and secondary health services, medication for depression and anxiety is very commonly prescribed and this may be the only input an individual receives. The medical model of mental illness is essentially pessimistic and offers little hope to service users. This is the case for a range of mental health problems, but particularly for personality disorder where enduring problems are central to the diagnosis and where it had traditionally been seen as untreatable.

However, in relation to major mental illness, literature from 1987 to 2003 identifies a number of long-term outcome studies which show upwards of 50 per cent recovery rates, or significant improvement over 20-year periods. Harding *et al.* (1987) suggest recovery levels of two-thirds of the people with major mental illness, such as schizophrenia, followed up over more than 30 years. In relation to personality disorder specifically, some treatments show good evidence of improved outcome. A meta-analysis of therapeutic communities, internationally, showed strong evidence for effectiveness across all 29 studies selected (Lees, Manning and Rawlings 1999). Perry, Banon, and Ianni (1999) conducted a meta-analysis of psychotherapy, drawing on literature from 1974 to 1998. Fifteen studies were selected and the analysis concluded that psychotherapy is an effective treatment for personality disorders and may bring about progress seven times faster than no treatment. The literature reflects further successful treatments for personality disorder at therapeutic communities and other specialist treatments as described below.

Psychological perspectives and treatments

Although personality disorder has dubious diagnostic validity within psychiatry, it does have a living meaning within mental health services. It also has a different meaning within the field of psychology where discourses between personality development and personality theory have been more closely linked. The value and benefits of a psychological approach in relation to understanding and treating personality disorder are described below.

Bowlby (1988), with regard to attachment theory and the concept of a secure base, describes how an individual tries to maintain proximity to another clearly identified person who is perceived as being able to cope better with the world and is expected to give care, comfort and security. This encourages us to value and continue relationships. Bowlby recognized that this attachment behaviour is emphasized in childhood but also continues throughout life. A child or adult who has attachment to someone is strongly disposed to stay near and seek contact with that individual, especially in times of threat and emergency. He observed that increased risk also carries a signal, for example, threats to abandon a child as a means of control, or parental threat of suicide. He suggested that this might also result in increased arousal, not just in terms of fear, but also intense anger, especially in older children or adolescents.

The dialectical theory of self-development assumes that a sense of self develops through the perception of oneself in another person's mind. An infant builds up a viable sense of self from the repeated internalization of the mother's processed image of the child's thoughts and feelings. This provides containment. Not only does the mother, or close care-giver, interpret the baby's physical expressions, she also gives back to the child a manageable interpretation of what is being communicated. Fonagy (1997) suggested that an absence, or distortion, of this early mirroring experience can lead to a desperate search on the part of the child to find alternative ways of containing psychological experience. This may develop into destructive physical expression, either towards self or others. A child who has not received recognized, but modified, images of behaviour and emotional states may have trouble in differentiating reality from fantasy and physical from psychic reality. This suggests a tendency, in later life, to cope with thoughts and feelings through physical action. Not being able to feel oneself from within, that individual is forced to find a sense of self from outside by treating themselves as an object or by getting others to react to them. This results in experience of self in a more authentic, if very limited, way and the need for re-enactment to augment the incomplete representation of self which has been achieved.

Herman and Van der Kolk (1987), in their work with incest victims and Vietnam veterans, discovered that trauma, especially prolonged trauma from care-givers, has a profound effect on personality development and the development of personality disorder. They concurred with Fonagy that behaviour manifestations of self-mutilation, re-victimization, victimizing others, dissociative disorders, substance abuse and eating disorders, are an effort to try to regain internal equilibrium. Van der Kolk (1996, p.3) has characterized this condition as *the black hole of trauma* and has described post-traumatic stress as a failure of time to heal all wounds. For some there is an inability to integrate the traumatic experience. He pointed out that there is a very complex interrelationship between trauma, neglect, environmental chaos and attachment patterns, and that clinicians fail to pay attention to the effects of early trauma or to perceive the patterns of reliving, warding-off reminders or repetitive re-exposure to situations reminiscent of trauma.

Bateman and Tyrer (2004), in their examination of psychological treatments for personality disorder, concluded that there was encouraging evidence that some patients were treatable but that there was inadequate evidence to make specific recommendations for any particular therapy. Psychological perspectives have given rise to a spectrum of specialist treatments for personality disorder involving both group work and individual therapy. A review of a range of therapies follows.

Dialectical behaviour therapy (DBT)

DBT was developed in the USA for the treatment of borderline personality disorder (Linehan 1993). When someone begins DBT there is an expectation that they will be committed to this therapy for at least a year. The program consists of a weekly, two-hour skills group and one-to-one therapy. The group aims to work together to achieve a life worth living. Dialectics involves finding the common ground between apparent opposites. In DBT this involves trying to balance positions that could be seen as contradictory, that is, accepting people as they are but also supporting them in change. The balance between acceptance and change is a central theme in DBT. Accepting people involves understanding that severe and enduring trauma has caused emotional vulnerability and a high sensitivity to life stresses. DBT involves a technique called mindfulness as well as other strategies which help the individual to learn to better tolerate distress and bear pain. The focus in DBT is on 'in the moment' skills, rather than dwelling on past trauma. It consists of four modules: *mindfulness*, which is a meditation approach that involves what, in DBT terms, is called taking hold of one's mind, meaning taking control of it; *interpersonal effectiveness skills*, which involves relationship skills, balancing priorities, 'shoulds' and 'wants' and self-concepts in relation to respect and competence; *emotion regulation*, involves learning to understand emotions, reducing vulnerability to them and decreasing emotional suffering; and *distress tolerance skills*, involving distracting, self-soothing and improving the moment. The first DBT randomized control trial compared DBT to treatment as usual (Linehan *et al.* 1991) and reported a drop in parasuicides and psychiatric inpatient stays, and better social adjustment. Feigenbaum (2007) highlights an emerging evidence base for the effectiveness of DBT revealed in four randomized controlled trials, again showing a reduction in parasuicidal behaviour, use of hospital bed days, in anger reduction and improvements in social functioning. In an article in the New York Times (2011) Dr Marsha Linehan, the creator of DBT, revealed that she had once been a service user, subject to sectioning, hospitalization and despair. Service users felt that the fact that Marsha had suffered herself from personality disorder went a long way to explain why she was able to develop such effective treatments.

Cognitive analytic therapy (CAT)

CAT is an integrative approach, used in the treatment of borderline personality disorder, utilizing cognitive behaviour and psychodynamic therapy (Ryle 1997). Here, the therapeutic value of the psychodynamic concepts of transference and counter-transference are recognized. The internalization of depriving and abusive care-givers results in a narrow or distorted range of what Ryle calls reciprocal roles. Examples of pair sets might include *abuser/abused, neglecting/deprived, controlling/rebellious* or *rejected/rejecting*. CAT therapists establish which aspect of the personality is maintaining dissociation and which particular contrasting self-state, or reciprocal role, the client uses to respond. Initial mapping of self-states is carried out collaboratively between therapist and client. The number of sessions may extend from 16 to 24 and a good outcome would be the internalization of the therapeutic relationship, enabling the client thereafter to become their own therapist. Denman (2001) highlighted that there was a growing, but still far from adequate, evidence base for the effectiveness of CAT. She suggested that there was a lack of randomized controlled trials validating CAT and that the supporters of RCT (randomized controlled trial) methodology tend to be less convinced by uncontrolled trials. Kerr (2006) highlights the educational effect of the CAT model on professionals and teams which was found to improve their containment of splitting and anxiety about clients. The therapeutic alliance was also found to reduce readmission rates during the course of therapy. The focus of Kerr's CAT study, therefore, differed in that it highlighted the systemic implications of working with personality disorder.

Schema therapy

Schema therapy (Young, Klosko and Weishaar 2003) combines elements of cognitive behavioural, emotion-focused, attachment and psychodynamic approaches. Its aim is to help clients to get their core needs met in an adaptive manner by working with early maladaptive schemas developed in childhood, when core needs were not met. Three schema driven coping styles are proposed: *schema surrender*, such as feeling and acting inadequate; *schema avoidance*, by suppressing feelings and avoiding situations which might evoke them; *schema overcompensation*, by striving or overworking in an attempt to counteract feelings of inadequacy. Jeffrey Young believes that many people with personality disorder have schemas which make traditional cognitive behaviour therapy (CBT) approaches unsuitable. Existing schemas might include self-sacrifice or approval seeking, feelings of abandonment and mistrust or shame, and an underdeveloped sense of self coupled with an unawareness of emotions and cognitions. This suggests that the addressing of such schemas should be the first step in therapy. Like DBT and CAT, schema therapy combines elements of other psychotherapies and approaches. It is usually a longer-term intervention of two to three years and, even for people with less severe difficulties, 20 sessions is rarely enough (Department of Health 2014). It was found to be highly effective in the first randomized controlled trial (Moran 2007). This randomized trial compared schema therapy with transference-focused therapy. Forty-six per cent of schema therapy patients made significant progress compared to 26 per cent of those engaged in transference focused therapy. They also showed greater increases in quality of life.

Transference-focused psychotherapy (TFP)

TFP consists of modified techniques grounded in psychoanalytic theory. Modifications are aimed to address the needs of people diagnosed with borderline personality disorder who have become split between the search for idealized and perfect care and their life experiences of abuse and neglect. Therapy begins with an explanation of what personality disorder is in terms of its being long-term and enduring rather than episodic. The person's internal sense of identity and difficulties with interpersonal relationships are also explored: emotions tend to be intense and rapidly shifting; relationships tend to be conflicted and stormy; there may be impulsive, self-destructive or self-defeating behaviours; and there is a lack of a clear and coherent sense of identity (Yeomans, Clarkin, and Kernberg 2002). Symptoms are also reviewed, some people may be impulsive and openly inappropriately angry, whereas others may have more internalized symptoms characterized by a sense of emptiness, fear of abandonment, suicidal feelings, and subtle shifts in their experience of others, ranging from idealizing others to feeling devalued by, or contemptuous of them. It is called transference-focused psychotherapy because the person is supported to explore their sense of self and others through observation of their experience of the therapy and the therapist. The aim of TFP is the integration of fragmented aspects of the personality which will enable the individual to establish good relationships and make commitments to life activities. In a randomized controlled trial examining TFP in relation to treatment by community psychotherapists (Doering *et al.* 2010), it was found that more people remained in therapy with TFP and that, although self-harming behaviour did not change in either group, significantly fewer in TFP attempted suicide, reducing the need for psychiatric in-patient treatment.

Mentalization therapy

Mentalization therapy techniques (Allen, Fonagy and Bateman 2006) have been developed for the treatment of borderline personality disorder and address the capacity to interpret the actions of ourselves and others on the basis of our own internal mental state. The capacity to interpret is developed in relation to our attachment experiences in early life. Acknowledging the fundamental vulnerability of someone with personality disorder, the model is based on Bowlby's attachment theory proposing that disrupted attachment relationships will result in a reduced capacity to mentalize. Fonagy and Bateman (2008) suggest that, during therapy, the vulnerability of clients means that they can easily be thrown into 'pretend mode'. They alert therapists to the importance of helping clients not to become over-identified by taking on the therapist's perspective as if it were part of themselves, but rather to focus on mental functions. This concerns addressing concreteness of thought and facilitating alternative perspectives.

Fonagy and Bateman also highlight the disruptive tendency of some clients to replicate unacceptable experiences with others by externalizing the abuser. Such projective identification can create emotionally unbearable conditions for a client. This needs to be addressed by a joint understanding of the therapist/client relationship that avoids over identification, and supports the client in learning to process roles and experiences. In a study carried out by Bateman and Fonagy (2008) 41 patients were engaged in a trial which compared mentalization-based treatment with treatment as usual. Findings showed that patients with 18 months of treatment, including partial hospitalization followed by mentalization-based group therapy, remained better than those receiving treatment as usual but that general social functioning remained impaired. Follow-up after five years showed that improvement in symptomatology was maintained.

Gans and Grohol (2010) cite the above therapies, dialectical behaviour therapy (DBT), schema therapy, transference-focused psychotherapy (TFP) and mentalization therapy as adapted psychotherapies that all address the underlying deficits in the ability of patients to manage emotions and relate to others, and which are proving successful for those who have longstanding problems stemming from childhood experiences. They suggest that recent trials do not show a consensus about whether any of these approaches prove most effective but note that DBT is the most widely taught.

Systems training for emotional predictability and problem-solving (Stepps)

The Stepps Group Program (Black *et al.* 2004) combines cognitive behaviour therapy (CBT) and schema therapy approaches and is considered to be adjunctive to other therapy someone is currently receiving. Here, two group leaders are CBT trained, a one-to-one reinforcer is available and a reinforcement team exists. The group program consists of 20 day sessions of two hours each, homework between sessions, one-to-one reinforcement from clinicians and an evening reinforcement team which can consist of family, carers and friends. The program includes a redefinition of borderline personality disorder to emotional intensity disorder; management strategies such as distraction and relaxation techniques; cognitive strategies that challenge unhelpful schemas; and behavioural strategies concerning problem-solving, abuse avoidance, lifestyle issues and goal setting. Members of the group have to be ready for therapy in terms of meeting certain criteria. They must be able to tolerate groups, have motivation, recognize there is a problem, be relatively un-chaotic and be free of severe problems that may interfere, such as substance misuse. The program originated in the USA (Blum *et al.* 2008) and has proven success for 53 clients in the six areas of Sussex where it has been established, with a further 25 who were still progressing in groups at that time. On six-month follow-up in Sussex, success was shown in dealing with the effects of trauma and in self-development, with a reduction in hospital bed usage and positive feedback from clinicians and service users (Harvey 2009).

Therapeutic communities

The therapeutic community model is a whole service model rather than a specific treatment. It involves a group of clients, sometimes referred to as residents, who have considerable involvement in running the community. There is recognition that service users are sometimes better able to assist each other than health professionals. The ability to flatten the hierarchy by delegating decision-making is still combined with firm leadership, while residents assume autonomy and responsibility for their own behaviour. Therapeutic communities are not just based on responsibility but also citizenship and empowerment (Campling 2001). Some therapeutic communities work only with psychodynamic groups while others include individual psychotherapy. All encourage the interest of members in learning about themselves and others, developing a culture of enquiry which constitutes a living, learning environment. Differing in structure from each other, therapeutic communities have a unifying philosophy that community can be used to contain its members while undergoing therapy. Haigh (1999) explains the five universal qualities which constitute a therapeutic environment: *attachment*, a culture of belonging; *containment*, a culture of safety; *communication*, a culture of openness; *involvement*, a culture of participation and citizenship; and *agency*, a culture of empowerment. Campling and Haigh (1999) extol the values of the therapeutic community model as a method of moving away from social control towards the development of therapeutic relationships and open-minded thinking.

Menzies, Dolan and Norton (1993) highlighted the economic importance of providing effective services for a client group that often consumes considerable amounts of psychiatric, social, probation and prison services in an unproductive way. Follow-up studies of 24 patients at the Henderson Hospital therapeutic community showed a saving of £12,700 per person, per year, meaning the cost of specialist treatment could be recouped in less than two years. The international review of studies about therapeutic communities mentioned earlier in this chapter, carried out by Lees *et al.* (1999), included 181 therapeutic communities in 38 countries. One hundred and thirteen of these therapeutic communities involved outcome studies, 52 of which were controlled and ten of which were randomized controlled trails. Twenty-nine acceptable studies emerged from a rigorous sifting process and strong evidence for effectiveness was shown across all 29 studies. Findings highlighted the effectiveness of the therapeutic community model in the treatment of personality disorder, particularly severe personality disorder.

The various approaches described above suggest that recovery may be possible. The National Institute for Health and Clinical Excellence, in addition to the new guidelines for borderline personality disorder (NICE 2009), has also issued guidelines for anti-social personality disorder (NICE 2010). The guidelines for anti-social personality disorder suggest that the evidence base for successful psychological treatments is limited (Duggan, Adams and McCarthy 2007) and that much more emphasis has been placed on psychological interventions for borderline personality disorder. Many treatments are mentioned in the borderline personality disorder guidelines, ranging from complimentary and art therapies to psychodynamic approaches, and they include all therapies mentioned above. Although the guidelines make brief mention that people with the diagnosis should be involved in planning personality disorder services, and that autonomy, choice, optimism and trust should be fostered, there is little more in the document that suggests a recovery ethos.

What is recovery?

Nehls (2000) suggested that, although some advances had been made, psychological approaches developed in treating personality disorder were not consistent with the concept of recovery as a vision constructed by the client and that a new vision of treatment, based on recovery, would require a fundamental shift in control from professionals to the person who is recovering. Therefore, it was essential in the second study to examine the underpinning values, in the field of mental health, in relation to the possibility of recovery and to identify the important factors in recovery for those diagnosed with personality disorder.

A history of recovery

Roberts and Wolfson (2006) place the origins of recovery-oriented care in this country, in the 18th century when William Tuke, a Quaker, developed a spiritual and family-like retreat in York. Here physical restraint was replaced by moral, psychological and work-oriented treatments in a safe and peaceful environment.

In the 19th century, John Percival wrote *A Patient's Account of his Psychosis, 1830 to 1832*, known as Percival's Narrative:

> *In the year 1830, I was unfortunately deprived of the use of reason …The Almighty allowed my mind to become a ruin under sickness – delusions of a religious nature, and treatment contrary to nature. My soul survived that ruin. (Percival 1961, p.3)*

This autobiographical account of mistreatment, and what actually helped, became an important forerunner of personal accounts about what is meaningful to recovery. This was followed, in more recent times, by the writings of people in the USA and UK. In the late 1980s a former service user with a diagnosis of schizophrenia first began to write about recovery as a new vision in mental health, encompassing hope and the challenge of living (Deegan 1988). In 1988, Judi Chamberlin wrote about her experiences in a landmark book called *On Our Own*. She made a compelling case for patient controlled services as an important alternative to public and private hospitals, which she believed had destroyed the confidence of so many. Other hope-inspiring accounts followed (Coleman 1999; Leete 1989; Reeves 1999; Unzicker 1989) accumulating a foundation of personal experiences relating to a recovery approach. These accounts concerned coping with symptoms, not being defined by illness and regaining a satisfactory sense of personal identity.

Professional rhetoric and international developments

By the late 1990s, The National Institute for Mental Health in England (NIMHE) introduced the concept of Mental Health Recovery as a central tenet of government policy and established the post of NIMHE Fellow for Recovery in 2000. In January 2005, NIMHE published a *Guiding Statement on Mental Health Recovery* which characterized recovery as the practice of values and the 'how' of service delivery and put service users at the heart of mental health recovery. Slade, Amering and Oades (2008) considered that this policy consensus became mirrored in professional rhetoric. In this country the concept of recovery was adopted by clinical psychology (British Psychological Society Division of Clinical Psychology 2000), mental health nursing (Department of Health 2006), occupational therapy (College of Occupational Therapists 2006) and psychiatry (Care Services Improvement Partnership, Royal College of Psychiatrists, and Social Care Institute for Excellence 2007). In the USA the term was adopted by the most internationally influential body in psychiatry (American Psychiatric Association 2005).

Canada, as well as Ohio and other US states, developed system performance indicators in relation to recovery (Brower 2003; Hogan 2001; Onken 2004; Roth *et al.* 2000). The Ohio eight-year longitudinal studies have shown that high concentration of service input has not necessarily lessened symptoms and that consumers considered themselves disempowered within the system. Therefore, core values of the Ohio initiative were that the concept of recovery should drive service provision and that, together, providers with consumers and their families should share responsibility for generating hope and determining services and supports. Outcome measures have balanced issues of access, quality and satisfaction with the practicalities of cost. Onken's study, based at Columbia University, New York, spanned nine US States. One of the primary findings of this study, considered integral to the process of recovery, was that mental health services must recognize and allow for self-agency while supporting such efforts and that the individual should be seen as a whole person beyond labelled identity. In 2000, concepts and policies related to recovery increased significantly in Australia (Slade *et al.* 2008). Australia was not only influenced by recovery literature from the USA and Canada, but also from New Zealand which, in 1998, became the first country to adopt a recovery ethos in mental health.

However, concurrent with this new vision, the existing psychiatric context still prevails, including diagnosis, prescribing and hospitalization. Hospitals may save lives, but Topor (2004) believes that the recovery context is simply not there in psychiatry and that the essence of the personal is destroyed within it. Topor relates a story about a secure ward outside Stockholm. After pressure from the psychology department, agreement was reached that the ward should be left unlocked. Somewhat to his disappointment no-one absconded for several weeks. One patient on the ward was a young Swedish girl who had been subject to both schizophrenia and personality disorder diagnoses at different times. Her demeanour was slow and lifeless, but one day she looked up and smiled at him and made a dash for the door. He describes running and running through the streets trying to catch up with her. She jumped into a train and he followed. When he reached her carriage he sat down and they began to engage in conversation and he discovered they had a mutual passion for art. They spent several hours in the city, looking through art galleries and at exhibitions, stopping for coffee to discuss what they had seen. Eventually he asked her if she thought they should return to the ward and she agreed, yes, it was okay to return now. Once back on the ward she returned to her slow and downcast demeanour. He tried to explain to staff how very changed she had been in a different context. However, the staff remained disbelieving.

Challenging the psychiatric context, recovery-oriented approaches in this country have included developments in the county of Devon. In 2003, the Wellness Recovery Action Plan, WRAP, developed by service users in the USA (Copeland 2001), was introduced to Devon. At its first small meeting in Exeter this recovery initiative became a group of peers where people were seen as just people rather than professionals or service users. The group was eventually launched as Recovery Devon and, since 2007, a top–down commitment to this bottom–up development resulted in the values and practical application of recovery principles being aspired to by commissioners and managers throughout mental health services in Devon. These values included a redefinition of what recovery means to those with severe mental health problems and opened the possibility of recovery to all (Roberts and Wolfson 2004).

Such initiatives have existed against a backdrop of less recovery-oriented services and this caused McGowan (2010) to question the concept of the 'expert by experience' as an NHS myth. He suggests that this is often of little or no use, resulting in tokenistic service user involvement, inviting fragmented and non-productive contributions, rather than the fundamental involvement of service users.

Defining recovery

Ramon, Healey and Renouf (2007) highlight that psychiatric services combine aspects of care and control whereas recovery oriented services shift responsibility to the individual service user. They suggest that governments who are preoccupied with risk management and reducing public funding may cause service users to fear that, if they are not 'recovering', services will no longer be available to them. Recovery as a clinical concept, measured in outcome studies as an approximation of cure, may be experienced as an imposition upon people struggling with serious and painful conditions, and as an unrealistic expectation and a burden to get well. Wallcraft (2005) considers that concerns, fears and objections to recovery will best be overcome by ensuring that it is a philosophy for life that becomes owned and defined by service users and survivors, and that this ownership must be respected by politicians, planners and service providers. Turner, Lovell and Brooker (2011) highlight the complexity of the recovery debate and how it has travelled a long way from its roots in the survivor movement. Here the emphasis for service users with a diagnosis of personality disorder has become one of self-discovery rather than recovery. They consider that the notion of recovery is a concept hijacked by mainstream services in a way which is unrealistic because it fails to acknowledge the challenges of living with the ongoing, painful legacy of trauma.

The word recovery has a range of meanings suggesting that conceptual clarity is necessary. Slade *et al.* (2008) identify two classes of meanings. First is the traditional concept of recovery as cure. This locates the concept within an illness framework. Second is the personal definition of recovery which has emerged from service user narratives. These accounts emphasize the understanding of recovery as something other than the absence of mental illness. Anthony (1993, p.16) proposes that the process of recovery can still take place in the presence of symptoms and disability, and defines recovery as:

> *A deeply personal, unique process of changing one's attitudes, values, feelings, goals, skills and roles. It is a way of living a satisfying, hopeful, and contributing life even with limitations caused by illness. Recovery involves the development of new meaning and purpose in one's life as one grows beyond the catastrophic effects of mental illness.*

Repper and Perkins (2003) suggest that recovery is not necessarily cure and is not about getting rid of all problems, but rather looking for the individual beyond problems and illness. Recovery may be a matter of finding abilities, possibilities, interests and dreams. It requires hope and opportunity. It is about building a future and recovering social roles and relationships that give meaning and value to life. Repper and Perkins see recovery as a process rather than a goal. Therefore recovery might best be defined as *the journey of recovery*.

There may be a risk in conceiving of recovery as a simple act of faith. However, recovery cannot be achieved without faith and hope (Roberts and Wolfson 2004). There is an assumption, in recovery oriented care, that professionals and clients will pursue client-oriented goals together, but decisions about what services are delivered are usually controlled by providers. Roberts and Wolfson suggest that, in contrast with a patient struggling for cure, recovery depends much more on collaboration than on treatment.

CHAPTER 3

The Journey Continues

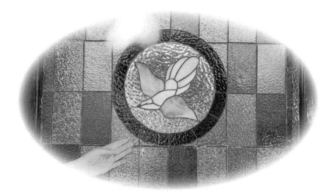

Isn't it about time professionals started to find out more about the realities of personality disorder and the self-destructive torment, frustration and utmost loneliness sufferers go through: Loneliness? Yes, loneliness because we are so misunderstood, humiliated, desperate and cut-off. Why, oh why, don't and won't these professionals accept that there is such a condition and illness? It is said that personality disorder cannot be treated. I think it can, with the help of different medications, but most of all by just sitting with us and recognizing and trying to understand this condition by listening.

Service User Quotation

For our local service users, being listened to, heard and understood was the aspiration, and the fulfilment of this desire was about to unexpectedly accelerate.

Linking with the national agenda

In 2002, during our period of disseminating the results of the earlier study in journal articles and at conferences, I was contacted by the Department of Health who had formed an expert group to create a National Personality Disorder Strategy. They were interested in our study and how they might meaningfully incorporate the views of service users within the strategy. I was invited to attend what I understood would be a meeting with the National Policy Head at the Department of Health. I arrived at Wellington House in London, long before its refurbishment. I was led down a rabbit warren of corridors and shown into a room with no windows. In this room, much to my astonishment, sitting around a large table were the members of the National Personality Disorder Strategy Group, here were some of the most famous names in the land, national authorities on personality disorder, names that we had actually quoted as references in our study. And here was I, an advocacy services manager from the 'boondocks' and they awaited my account of research efforts in North East Essex.

After listening to my description of our collaborative service user study, the Strategy Group decided to hold a series of focus groups and it was planned that these groups would involve service users with a personality disorder diagnosis from different parts of the country, including members of our group. Their views were to have a significant impact on national strategy (Haigh 2003). On 23 January, 2003, new National Guidance, *Personality Disorder: No Longer a Diagnosis of Exclusion* (Department of Health 2003a), was launched. We considered ourselves to be significant stakeholders in the new guidance because we believed that our service user research work in North East Essex had a bearing on the development of the national agenda in relation to personality disorder.

Within this meaningful development, concerns about funding for needed services remained. However, by the middle of the year the *Personality Disorder Capabilities Framework, Breaking the Cycle of Rejection* (Department of Health 2003b) was being created with a view to addressing national training needs regarding the diagnosis. I attended a meeting about this training strategy, again at Wellington House. It is true that clouds can have silver linings because, in the midst of fears regarding a revised Mental Health Act potentially introducing new and repressive legislation, the Department of Health began to talk about investment in pilot projects for service delivery and workforce training. Complete with this bit of intelligence, I dashed back to Essex and rounded up our service user group

41

to tell them the news. Our local research had given clues to better service response, ranging from being listened to, understood and feeling safe, to an out-of-hours helpline, a safe house and a crisis house. However, at this meeting of the local Personality Disorder Group in Colchester in June 2003, the service users now began to explore, in earnest, what ingredients would comprise a service that could really meet their needs. They had a long wish list and a very clear idea of what they considered was required and this is what they had to say:

We need more communication – no one talks to you.

The response is too slow.

We don't want to be told we're not ill.

We need acceptance and staff who understand.

We need a relaxed atmosphere where we are respecting one another and we have peer support.

The day hospital isn't always the right place for us, and nor is the acute ward.

Some of us need substance abuse help and they don't understand it here.

We need help in a crisis.

We need a Crisis House and crisis support.

We need help to prevent suicide attempts.

We can feel very unsupported and need help earlier.

We need mentoring/buddying.

A befriending service.

One-to-ones.

Groups can be too deep for us.

We need groups when we are ready:

    talking groups

    writing groups

    craft groups

    some service user-led groups.

We need education in:

>   positive thinking
>
>   coping strategies
>
>   anger management.

We need practical help with:

>   advocacy
>
>   benefits
>
>   housing
>
>   child protection issues
>
>   legal/criminal justice support.

We like the idea of alternative therapies:

>   massage
>
>   acupuncture
>
>   reflexology.

Don't forget gay and lesbian support.

43

We need the right kind of therapies to be available:

>   CBT
>
>   CAT
>
>   DBT
>
>   counselling and psychotherapy.

We need all services to be working together:

>   medication if we need it
>
>   CPA (the care program approach)
>
>   a strong link to statutory services.

We need a secure base where we are understood and where we can help each other, where we can get help in a crisis 24/7, and where we can get and give ongoing support.

The national proposals called for eight service pilots throughout England, one for each region of the country. We were inspired and eager to submit a tender to be one of the national pilot projects. Our next step was to create a multi-stakeholder group which would work to compile a pilot proposal for our area. Members of our local personality disorder group joined with representatives from other local service user groups and Colchester Mind, the local Mental Health Trust, local Primary Care Trusts, Housing Providers, the Borough Council, the Accident and Emergency Department and Essex Police.

The Haven was chosen as a working name for the proposal. Local service users liked the title and the name stuck because it seemed to embody everything we were trying to achieve. The proposal for The Haven was created entirely around the service users' views outlined above. Our service users flanked the proposal every step of the way. This began with their presentations at the National Institute of Mental Health Eastern Development Centre where we made it through the second round of selections.

The service user focus groups held at national level were now transformed into a National Personality Disorder Service User Reference Group and some of our local service users joined. This Group of 'experts by experience' worked in parallel with the National Expert Personality Disorder Group to select the successful pilot projects. Local service user members of the group were, of course, asked to declare an interest when proposals for The Haven were tabled for consideration. I knew all service users involved had been sworn to secrecy regarding proceedings. When our local service users returned from London after one of their meetings I met them at the advocacy office and made it clear that I would not try to elicit any information from them. One of the service users smiled and then swung a rucksack off her back, revealing that she had actually brought a bag full of information! Stolen goods? Would a breach of protocol ever be discovered? But looking at this unexpected bounty was hard to resist and we pored over the proposals from different regions which were impressive in many different ways. However, our service users said that, at the London meeting, the other service users had rated The Haven as the top desirable service design in the country. Although we did not have information regarding the views of the professionals from the National Expert Personality Disorder Group, our hopes began to run high.

Eleven service pilots were chosen, one was selected for each region of England apart from London, which had three, and Eastern Region, where two were selected, one being The Haven. The news came in February 2004. There was an explosion of excitement amongst both our service users and local mental health professionals. One psychiatrist said to me, 'Now the headaches begin!', and it was true that amongst all the jubilation I also felt extremely daunted at the prospect of actually having to create this new project which we had dreamed of for so long. By the middle of the year we began to create the new local service.

First days at The Haven

The service was launched on 1 June 2004, as a voluntary sector organization with many stakeholders. This included important representation from the local Mental Health Trust who leased us temporary premises. This had been the home of a former day hospital housed in the old Railway Mission in Colchester, an interesting building which we loved with its high gothic-like ceilings, which would enable us to have the tallest ever Christmas tree for our first Haven Christmas. The multi-agency group we had formed to create our pilot proposal now comprised The Haven Steering Group and ten members were drawn from it to form a Board of Directors, five of whom had used mental health services. I had spent some weeks putting together an Operational Policy and many other attendant, crucial policy documents which had to be newly created because, being a voluntary sector project, we could not take advantage of existing policy documents in the statutory domain. Organizationally, we were starting from nothing. On that first day of June in 2004 our Chairman unpacked the boxes containing our computers and I was the sole staff member. We began to recruit, with service users on every interview panel, and we soon had administrative staff. Excited service users were 'storming the doors' to be registered and, while recruiting the day staff, I began to register the first clients of The Haven. Together with our administrator and some of our clients, we opened a Friendship Group on Tuesday afternoons to accommodate service user need, and the enthusiasm of all, to make a start.

In June 2004 we held our first Research Group Meeting where we began to discuss ideas for a second research study with the initial aim of looking at whether The Haven Project was effective over the two years of the proposed pilot period. This would be a natural follow-up of previous local research. There would be training for service user researchers and payment would be made within the confines of the therapeutic earnings limits. The minutes of this meeting are included at the beginning of the Research Diary, Appendix II. Ideas for the new service also proliferated at this first meeting: homely; normal; common ground; a problem-free room; the golden phone call; a Sweetie Shute. The latter idea was responded to during our first months by the ever-present bowl of chocolate sweeties at The Haven. Present, that is, until our finance officer presented me with a total of all we had spent on chocolates over those first few weeks, suggesting a bit more prudence. It is true, however, that chocolate did somehow become an ongoing theme at The Haven during my ten-year tenure and our home baked cakes were described as 'legend'.

During the summer of 2004 I met with Shula Ramon, then Professor of Inter-professional and Social Studies at Anglia Ruskin University, who had been my principle supervisor for the initial research study which, academically, had constituted an MA dissertation. The funding proposal for The Haven included a research budget and discussion with Professor Ramon concerned how the earlier research study about personality disorder could be continued by building research structures into the new service, and how it could be supported academically as a PhD study. Earlier research had examined the nature of the diagnosis and the way in which it was responded to by psychiatric and other services. The Haven would provide a new service context where support and treatment could now be examined.

It was agreed by all that the research events for the study would begin when we moved to our permanent home, at Glen Avenue in Colchester, and opened all parts of the service. The Glen Avenue premises had been used as an eight-bedded half-way house for people being discharged from psychiatric hospital into the community, again owned by the local Mental Health Trust. It was due to close down. As an advocate I might more usually have been 'agitating' about the fact that the Mental Health Trust was closing one of its service areas. However, its availability was most opportune and, while I might have briefly considered my dichotomy of responsibilities, in truth we were easily suborned by this bit of payola and we were more than grateful that it was being leased to us.

Whilst engaged in two days of recruitment for staff to man the out-of-hours crisis service, we received a call from the Ward Councillor, who happened to live across the back garden wall to our proposed home in

Glen Avenue. The spirit of her call was one of determined opposition. I had not applied to the Borough Council Planning Office for change-of-usage as the building was to continue to be used for mental health purposes. However, there would be many more clients and specifically clients diagnosed with personality disorder. When the local Councillors discovered the plan they were dismayed. A well-attended meeting was held one Saturday morning at the Ward Councillor's home. Many local people from the area participated and they were clearly concerned about the impact of The Haven on such a lovely neighbourhood. We suspected house values might have also figured in concerns. While awaiting this meeting we did not know what to expect or how much hostility we might encounter. I attended the meeting with our Chairman and one of our service users who spoke bravely and compellingly about her past and the need for our planned service. This moved one neighbour to tears and she made a lovely statement on behalf of the local church, who became firm supporters of The Haven thereafter.

We were now required, of course, to apply for planning permission for The Haven. This delayed all plans for moving to our permanent home and opening the remaining parts of the project. We were half way through recruiting staff for the out-of-hours part of the service. We needed to make a decision about what to do next. Again the Mental Health Trust was more than helpful and the Area Director gave her permission to open the out-of-hours crisis phone line and to allow clients to be present out-of-hours at our temporary premises.

The phone lines buzzed from the word go. However, clients attending out-of-hours presented high distress and risk. For weeks it became the norm to accommodate them overnight on armchairs and couches. When I arrived each morning I used to step over the sleeping to water the plants. It was a health and safety nightmare akin to a doss house and the new Board of Directors of The Haven was up in arms.

I attended the planning meeting with two of our service users in January 2005 and we were granted planning permission initially for one year. So…we were on license to prove our good behaviour. Planning issues were the beginning of many and varied battles and challenges over the years to keep The Haven on an even keel and flourishing. We were at great pains to prove ourselves to the neighbourhood. We held events and strawberry teas and became involved in the local Open Gardens initiative with St Leonard's Church. The church also helped us by loaning the junior church choristers at Christmas time each year. This enabled us to hold very

47

special carol services for the local community. We created a Being Good Neighbours policy with leaflets and posters. Cursing in the garden became a treasonous offence and, in fact, making any kind of disturbance outside was likely to bring The Haven Community down on one like a ton of bricks because Haven clients held our good name in the neighbourhood in such high regard.

The following year we were granted three-year's planning consent, and three years later our consent became permanent. By this time we had made friends and allies of the neighbours and our Ward Councillor had long ago given her apologies for her initial response to The Haven and became a firm supporter throughout her Mayor-ship and continuation as Ward Councillor. Again, I attended this final planning meeting with our clients and we made our way, for the third time, to the ancient and opulent rooms of Colchester Town Hall. The Planning Committee gave its consent, with a codicil concerning their regret that The Haven had been put through such unnecessary scrutiny over the years. Their statement ended with some final words about this client group obviously not being one that causes any kind of trouble in the community. I thought, 'Blimey, we've overdone it!'

Planning consent was preceded by a flurry of activity to create our new home in the way that we wanted it to be. The old stained glass front door had been shattered by someone's stray rocket on November 5th fireworks night, weeks before we moved in, and one of our clients took on the long task of recreating a beautiful new stained glass panel with a dove at its centre. National Mind had recently, and to my sadness, decided to forgo the white dove as its symbol. We decided the white dove would now be the symbol of The Haven. The tale of how the stained glass door was restored is included in Chapter 8, from the perspective of Dee who carried out this wonderful piece of work. Our next task was to clear rooms. Two more clients, Pablo and Cosmic, set to work. They relished smashing up a number of old wardrobes surplus to our requirements; very satisfying and legitimate delinquency. Afterwards I stood outside with Pablo looking up at the building in Glen Avenue, which we felt was so beautiful and so suited to our needs. We had a moment of hysteria at the thought that it was now ours; a sense of unreality; a 'rags to riches' story.

Together with service user volunteers, we cleaned and we had painters redecorate throughout. We moved furniture, hung pictures, placed plants and shelved books. By the end of three weeks, fatigue had reduced our task force to one service user and me. We were exhausted and our administrator and finance officer took pity and swooped in like the 'Fifth Cavalry' to hang curtains, make beds and plump new cushions. The results felt wonderful and on 31 January 2005, we moved to Glen Avenue, our permanent premises, and opened all parts of the service.

Service context for our new study

The Haven aspired to be a sanctuary with a sense of safety, wholeness, caring and home which was a place of refuge and protection (Bloom 1997). Housed in an old Rectory in Colchester, with 18 rooms, within its walls the décor was warm and inviting and the artwork was largely painted by clients, its peaceful atmosphere spreading to the boundaries of its garden.

The services offered included a therapy and group program from Monday to Friday, 24-hour crisis phone and text lines and a Safe Centre where those in crisis could come for a few hours, at any time of the day or night, on any day of the week. There were also four bedrooms, which constituted a Crisis House, where people could find respite from outside pressures for one night or up to three weeks.

People diagnosed with personality disorder often experience high anxiety states born of chronic hyper-arousal. Therefore, we believed that such a sanctuary should provide a relaxed, de-escalating environment where a range of options would be available such as companionship, information, creative and distracting activities and groups, being able to talk to staff about difficulties and safely express emotions at any time of the day or night, life skills lessons and more structured therapy. It included complementary therapies to help soothe the kinds of anxiety symptoms experienced physically as well as mentally. It encouraged humour as a form of shared intimacy, promoting laughter and allowing playfulness that would help to recapture a healthy sense of being a child. This included activities like The Haven Hat Society which met at 12.37½ pm on Thursdays, in the parlour, to discuss such topics as the benefits and pitfalls of extreme hat-wearing. 'Tea and tiffin are provided if we can be bothered.' Hats ranged from towel-turbans to yashmaks, with many eccentric variations in-between.

The Haven would be not just a physical setting, but a unique aspiration to create a sanctuary which was peaceful and accepting and which belonged to its service users. With its non-institutional aura it stood outside the norm for mental health service settings and was the antithesis of what can be the bleak prospect of an NHS environment.

Rationale for the new study

In the 1990s, the grounds for the earlier study sprang from the awareness that the diagnosis of personality disorder was being treated separately and differently. At this time there was an absence of real efforts to understand the difficulties of those who had attracted the diagnosis or to provide services that met their needs. The prevailing climate suggested not only that personality disorder was enduring but, additionally, that it was intractable and likely to be untreatable. The earlier inquiry (Castillo 2003) yielded a new understanding of the diagnosis, defined by those with a personality disorder, and contributed to a change in the national agenda when the Department of Health responded in 2003 by providing national guidance and funding for pilot projects throughout the country. This resulted in The Haven, the service context for a new study.

The Haven was a new service which had been set up with the intention of meeting needs, but to what degree would it do so and to what extent would it be successful in effecting social inclusion for clients with a personality disorder diagnosis? Internationally, there was no agreed rationale of recovery for those diagnosed with personality disorder and few researchers had sought the views of service users regarding this (Stalker, Ferguson and Barclay 2005). Roberts and Wolfson (2004) emphasized the need to develop research methods that incorporate subjective accounts of recovery from service users in order to better inform professionals, and suggested that professionals would find little guidance about what might help recovery from a medically-oriented randomized controlled trial. Examination of the psychotherapeutic, social and material aspects of the process of recovery was needed from the perspective of those with a diagnosis of personality disorder. This is what the new study set out to do.

50

CHAPTER 4

The Research Journey

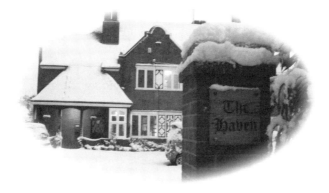

People found their voices because of the research, where they hadn't found them before. Being part of this research group I learned that we were really being listened to and I actually saw the changes being made in response to what we said and things have moved on in a measurable way. It's not just a learning curve about the research project, it's about how we've all changed and grown.

Service User Quotation

We had moved to our new home at the end of January and it was now February 2005. The four beds of the Crisis House were opened and the service began to move into a calmer and more settled pattern. I have long believed that, as human beings, thriving is our default setting. Up to now this had not proven to be the case for our clients, who bore a sense of self-fracture and fragmentation. However, the homeliness and peacefulness of The Haven and the sense of hope that permeated the air had an effect on all of us. In those early days at The Haven we believed that we were unlikely to achieve change by fighting the existing reality. Our aim was to change things by building a new model that could even make the old ways obsolete (Fuller 2002).

The Research Group begins

The Research Group was a prime mover in our research journey. As mentioned in the last chapter, the group was formed in June 2004 and it met until September 2009. Appendix II is a Research Group Diary which constitutes a précis of the minutes of 35 Research Group meetings occurring during that time. The Research Diary gives the inside story in detail and reveals the participatory nature of the second study. The group essentially consisted of ten core members, me and nine Haven clients.

A crucial concern for Research Group members, at their first meeting, was that *recovery* was not a term they would have chosen. They set out to define recovery in their own terms. Recovery implies returning to a previous state of being, whereas members were seeking to create a new future, the future they wanted, and maybe to become reborn, not to go back to all that was wrong in the first place. Our concept of the length of the study was modest at the outset. We aimed to look at whether, how, and why The Haven was successful over its first two years and we expected to apply for ethical permission to conduct the research within a few short months.

In order to achieve valid results in the research we understood that, academically, it needed to adhere to certain methodologies. This would help to assure credibility for our results. It was also important to us to have a logical and reasoned approach to our task that would be consistent with our humanistic ideals. Following is a description of our approach, methods and how we carried out the research.

Research questions

We set out to explore and understand, from the service user perspective, the process of recovery for people diagnosed with personality disorder, using The Haven as a case study. The aim of the study was to find answers to the following questions:

- How do those with a personality disorder diagnosis define recovery?

- What factors are important in taking control over one's life for those diagnosed with personality disorder?

- Does The Haven, as a project, contribute to this process, and if so how?

Philosophical approach

One major philosophical approach to research is the scientific interpretation of data that can be directly observed. It pursues scientific awareness which records only directly observed phenomena, and opinions are claimed to be untrustworthy (Kolakowski 1995). This approach to the pursuit of knowledge has contributed to great developments in science and technology, and this philosophy of human inquiry held sway throughout the 19th and 20th centuries, and maintains a dominant influence in the sciences today. Here, researchers would be concerned with numbers of people attracting a diagnosis of personality disorder, percentages receiving certain treatments or no treatment, and numbers subject to hospitalization, for example.

A second and alternative approach, which began to gain prominence at the end of the 19th century, rejects the above philosophy as the single ideal for the rational understanding of reality (Hammersley 1989). Consistent with this alternative approach is the philosophy of *hermeneutics* which is a term derived from the wing-footed Greek God Hermes, the messenger of the Gods, the bringer of wisdom. Hermeneutics is concerned with human behaviour rather than with physical phenomena (Rowan and Reason 1981). Here human beings are considered to have the ability to give meaning to their experience. This opens the door to an interpretive approach, with an emphasis upon the description of reality through the eyes of participants.

Using another winged creature as an analogy, these different approaches to the gleaning of knowledge might be understood by considering the birds. A scientific study might be made about birds, their habitats, feeding and other factors. However, if we could speak to the birds they might tell us so much more. They might tell us that Mrs Brown offers a particularly good quality of breadcrumbs on her lawn, hence the reason why so many blackbirds congregate and thrive in her garden. The wrens might tell us that it is not just about the nesting quality of the vegetation at the bottom of Mr Green's garden but the fact that the Greens play soft music in their garden pergola, music that the wrens just love to chirp along to. Who knows what they might tell us and, taking this one step further, what

53

might we find out if a bird was to talk to the other birds, in bird-speak as it were, and bring back another layer of meaning to us. This would be a kind of *double-hermeneutics*, where the researchers try to make sense of the participants making sense of their world (Smith 2003). This, therefore, was the philosophical approach we chose as a way to explore reality through the eyes of participants in order to interpret the deeper meanings in their lives.

The participative dimension

Freire (1970) suggested that the study of a problematic or oppressive reality should not be carried out by experts but by those experiencing the oppression.

> *It is only the oppressed who, by freeing themselves, can free their oppressors. The latter, as an oppressive class, can free neither others nor themselves. It is therefore essential that the oppressed wage the struggle to resolve the contradiction in which they are caught. (Freire 1970, p.10)*

This process of mutual learning is achieved through a creative dialogue between researcher and participant, or co-researchers, which seeks meaning and change.

> *Human existence cannot be silent nor can it be nourished by false words, but only by true words, with which men and women transform the world. To exist humanly is to name the world, to change it. (Freire 1970, p.34)*

Therefore, words would be our touchstone. Not for us the medically oriented approach of a randomized controlled trial. Rather, by participation, by a Conference of the Birds (Attar 1984), we would seek meaning.

Participatory action research (PAR) is a way of conducting research which is designed and carried out by all participants, including the initiating researcher. It focuses on concerns highlighted by the reflections of those involved (Winter and Munn-Giddings 2001). Most research serves those in power, such as governments or managers (Stanton 1989) and researching those who comprise stigmatized groups can be a form of oppression (Gorman 1999). Therefore, a central issue in participatory action research is empowerment and its goal is democratic as well as collaborative. It challenges inequality and establishes the right of people to actively participate in processes that affect their lives. Some researchers

54

advocate that, wherever possible in the field of disability, service users should become researchers, with control over the selection of issues to be researched, data collection, analysis and dissemination (Evans and Fisher 1999).

A participatory action research approach was selected for the study because it recasts the roles of researcher and participant. It provides a vehicle where both the initiating researcher and all those participating can come to see the problem in a radically different way, which may give rise to innovative action for change. In the second study there were a relatively large number of participants who had a variety of roles and different power in relation to the endeavor. Most were members of a stigmatized group who had attracted a diagnosis of personality disorder and all became involved in some way in the cyclical spiralling process of change which begins with dialogue about the problem, collectively generated solutions for change, putting those changes into action, and reflections and evaluations of those changes from which lessons can be learned and more changes generated.

Methods used in the research

Quantitative methods in research are essentially numerical and objectively observable. They are concerned with frequency, averages and percentages that can be analyzed by statistical methods (Fuller and Petch 1995). Such studies ask 'How much?'; 'How often?'; 'What percentage?' and 'What proportion?' However, the *quantitative* approach excludes rich veins of knowledge, understanding and potential for change (Bannister *et al.* 1994). Rowan and Reason (1981) criticize this method as lacking in social context, alienating and disempowering, detached and dehumanizing. Nevertheless, because quantitative data is in a numerical form it can be more easily presented graphically and can be used to compare tendencies in populations and between groups. Such scientific approaches are a major contributor to the descriptions of personality disorder in the Diagnostic and Statistical Manual of Mental Disorders, DSM 5, and its European counterpart, ICD 10, which focus on surface manifestations and not the experiences of the sufferer. However, we considered that in a study such as this, which would be rich in subjective experience, the statistical tables provided by quantitative approaches should not be ruled out as they might strengthen the research data by describing aspects of it in numerical terms.

The *qualitative* approach is the interpretive study of a particular issue or problem (Parker 1994). Qualitative research is part of a debate rather than a fixed truth. It uses data in the form of words rather than numerical information. It is an attempt to capture the reality that lies within by using verbal data, which highlights depth and meaning rather than reducing it to numerical scores. It involves building rapport and credibility with participants and the employment of methods that are humanistic and interactive.

The qualitative approach begins with participants' views, which are then interpreted by the researcher and can encompass interaction and a complexity of perspectives. This approach was chosen because we believed it would provide the most effective method for collecting data which can be described and interpreted. It accommodated the emancipatory style of participatory action research where participants would also be researchers involved in both descriptions and interpretations.

The methods of data collection included focus groups and individual interviews, which are described below. The methods of data collection and analysis are represented in a Timeline in Appendix I which also gives a chronology of all aspects of the research endeavor.

Focus groups are a meeting of a small group of people who are facilitated through a discussion relevant to the research. Participants are asked about their opinions and perceptions in relation to a service or an idea. Such a group can reveal hidden aspects of problematic life experiences in a dynamic and empowering way (Padilla 1993). Focus groups are a collective method of meaning-making and can be taped and transcribed to create a full account of what is said. A major risk in this method is that participants may respond, within the pressure of a group situation, in ways that lack fidelity to their actual experiences and opinions (Zeller 1993). The research agenda and questions can achieve a mitigation of such risks by repetitively addressing themes from different perspectives. Problems can also arise in relation to one or more respondents dominating the discussion. Boundaries and guidelines, made clearly known to participants from the outset and the facilitator's vigilance in addressing such issues during discussion, are likely to minimize such occurrences.

Individual interviews were not a method originally considered for data collection. This would mean separating interactions from others because the dialogue would occur between interviewer and individual interviewee which did not seem consistent with the approach which had been adopted for the study. The Research Group, focus groups and other groups at The Haven invited a multitude of interpersonal dynamics to occur. Participatory and collaborative research begins and ends in shared activities and understanding, captured in the dialogue of groups, as the main method of revealing all participants to themselves (Padilla 1993). However, we discussed the possibility that individual interviews with some participants might provide additional dimensions of data possibly more easily disclosed in a private setting.

Whittaker (2009) considers the effective use of focus groups for accessing shared public knowledge, compared to the fruitful setting of individual interviews for highlighting more personal and biographical data. He suggests that interviews can be used, in conjunction with focus groups, to access sensitive information that might not arise in a group setting. Creswell (2003) also suggests that individual questionnaires or interviews can be legitimate in a participatory action research approach to generate information that could not be ascertained in another way. This was considered by the Research Group and it was decided that it would be an additional, valuable dimension of data collection which should be encompassed.

Collecting the data

By January 2005 a stable membership of the Research Group had formed, however, before we could begin holding focus groups we needed to refine our research questions and gain ethical permission for the study. In the interim, we were enthusiastic about a plan to hold *service evaluation groups* (SEGs) which would give us the opportunity to test and refine research questions and would help everyone to become familiar with this kind of forum. The date for the first *service evaluation group* (SEG) was set for February 2005, which was just days after we moved to our permanent premises at Glen Avenue and opened all parts of the service. There was a great sense of excitement about the first research event and about the stories that needed to be told. There was a curiosity about others and a sense of valuing how important each individual was within their own narrative. There was also a commitment from participants to informing the development of The Haven in all its aspects. We wanted to include anyone who was interested in participating and ensured that all clients registered at The Haven would receive an invitation to the first SEG by posters and mailings. With the permission of attendees, it was agreed that the SEGs should be taped to enable full transcripts of what was said to be made available. At the Research Group meeting in March 2005 members felt that the SEG had been a great success. From the outset it was a dynamic and fascinating forum with constructive criticism and a highlighting of improvements to be implemented. The honesty and laughter were appreciated and it was agreed that SEGs should be held every three months until formal data collection began. Creation and refinement of research questions continued at the SEGs and the final SEG Questionnaire is included as Appendix III to give a flavour of the types of questions that were asked.

The second supervisor from our earlier study, Dr Nicola Morant, had joined Professor Shula Ramon at Anglia Ruskin University in Cambridge, meaning that the old academic team had reformed. University supervisors suggested that participants should have pseudonyms, enabling us to distinguish between respondents and to see development over time.

At the April 2005 meeting of the Research Group, after a discussion about barriers to recovery, the group decided to add a question about whether or not recovery is frightening, which proved crucial for gleaning rich data. Thirteen clients attended the second SEG in May 2005 and, at the July 2005 Research Group meeting, it was agreed that questions for future SEGs should remain the same because this would provide a consistent yardstick. From this time SEG questions remained as they are shown in full in the SEG Questionnaire (Appendix III). Until ethical permission for the study was requested and granted, and formal data collection was begun, four more SEGs were held until May 2006. This was a total of six SEGs taking place at three-monthly intervals. The Research Group also considered that, after completion of the focus groups, the SEGs should resume at regular intervals and two more were held before the end of the study, in August and November 2007.

Research supervisors at the university considered that the facilitation of focus groups, and the conducting of individual interviews, should be carried out by a service user participant rather than by me, because I was also Chief Executive at The Haven. Therefore, the Research Group was tasked with selecting one of its members to be the service user researcher, who would facilitate focus groups and carry out individual interviews, in the more formal phase of data collection. This highlighted a possible dilemma in that more than one service user may have wanted to take up this role. The group may not have reached agreement about who should do this and may have wished to select someone that they felt comfortable with but about whom I had reservations, in terms of intellectual grasp and ability to draw out themes. One member wished to take up the role and, fortunately, we all felt she met the various necessary criteria. She had previous research experience, was educated and warm, and the unanimous decision of the group suggested that she was someone to be trusted both academically and emotionally. Payment was also agreed for each attendance by participants at a research event and also additional payment for each event that the service user research facilitator conducted.

The intention of the Research Group was to use the SEG questions in Appendix III as focus group questions. However, university research supervisors suggested refinements regarding wording and sequence. At the Research Group meeting in April 2006, members felt it was important to retain current questions but to be open to small adjustments. At the June 2006 meeting members agreed the final draft of focus group questions compiled from the suggestions of academic supervisors. A more logical order was achieved, questions were less leading and opportunities had been added to explore the impact of The Haven as a therapeutic community. This agreement regarding amendments came with the exception of question six which concerned disliking oneself less. Suggested revision from university supervisors tabled a more straightforward question about liking oneself more. The group considered that the double-negative phrasing of the original question was more conducive to eliciting valid answers from people with personality disorder. With me acting as go-between this process represented an interesting dialogue between client participants, who conceived of the questions, and academic supervisors, who added their research expertise for final question formulation. The Research Group's refusal to change question six represented their empowered position regarding what they felt was right and the fact that this was their research. To me the double-negative question was one that was inspired by those who had received the diagnosis and it made me smile to think that probably only they could have conceived of it. It was another highly successful question in practice. This became question seven in the client focus group questions, which were then finalized and are included here as the Focus Group Questionnaire, Appendix IV.

Focus groups seemed a natural progression from the service evaluation groups (SEGs), which had yielded so much information in the previous year and a quarter. The focus group method also proved to be a dynamic form of data collection where one participant's thoughts and ideas might spark and elicit responses from others. Maintaining a three-monthly rhythm, the timetable (Appendix I) reflects a seamless change from the last service evaluation group in May 2006, to the first client focus group in August 2006. Four client focus groups were held, at three-monthly intervals, the fourth taking place in May 2007. Each focus group was one and a half hours long and all clients were invited by advertising, with posters and mailings, and attendance was by self-selection. The focus groups were similar in flavour to the SEGs, with use of pseudonyms and transcribed tapes, but attendance was limited to a maximum of 12 in order to ensure significant time and space for all participants. Some continuity of attendance for participants was maintained at focus groups to aid mapping of experiences and progress over time. Participants came for a variety of reasons ranging from curiosity to the sense of empowerment achieved in articulating views and listening to the views of others. Because some attended all or most focus groups, this provided an opportunity to reflect on progress over time. Those who had also attended the SEGs provided additional mapping over a two and three-quarter year period.

The Research Group constructed a Client Interview Questionnaire that contained an interview schedule which mirrored the client focus group questions. Because it was considered that there would be more time and space during individual interviews, an additional question about comparison with other services was added. Two questions about The Haven as a community were also added, one of which was also included in the focus group questions. It was agreed that the wording and the sequence of the interview schedule would be consistent with the changes suggested by supervisors for the client focus group questions. Preceding the interview schedule were a series of tick box questions which would help to profile the sample. The Client Interview Questionnaire is shown as Appendix V.

It was anticipated that interviews were likely to be approximately one hour long, which proved to be the case, and it was agreed that they should be taped and transcribed. Twenty interviews were considered to be the number we should conduct in relation to other data collection occurring in the study. It was judged that this number would encompass a range of clients from the service and they were conducted between August 2006 and July 2007. Some participants attended focus groups as well as individual interviews and results reflected that different dimensions of information arose in an alternative setting. Other participants for interviews were suggested by the Research Group. Some of the clients suggested by the group had found it more difficult to participate in SEGs and in focus group activities and readily agreed to be interviewed on an individual basis because they considered it would be a more palatable setting in which to disclose sensitive information. I continued to attend group research events as a silent participant but did not attend individual interviews. Therefore, the data came to me and the Research Group after completion of each interview, however, the content of the interviews was no less rich and exciting to read than hearing participant accounts first-hand at the focus group events.

The involvement of carers and family members in the study was discussed at the Research Group meeting in January 2006. Academic supervisors also considered that carers and family members were logical partners in this inquiry because of their close association with the day to day living of clients. It was decided that two carer focus groups would be held and the Research Group drafted their ideas for the questionnaire. Proposed interview questions were circulated to eight carers for comments and refinement. The carer focus group questions are shown as Appendix VI. It was important to reflect on the burden of personality disorder from a relative or carer's perspective and if and how The Haven impacted on this. An examination of carers' perspectives about recovery were also considered as a point of comparison with service users' views and to ascertain to what degree hope was present. The carer focus groups invited up to ten participants by mailings via all Haven clients and attendance was by self-selection, with prior agreement of the client concerned. Carer focus groups were one and half hours long and were also taped and transcribed. Someone who was a carer for a Haven client was selected as facilitator for the carer focus groups. This choice was approved by the Research Group and again it was suggested that this person met both empathic and intellectual criteria. She facilitated both carer focus groups, which were held in March and August 2007.

The Research Group was essentially concerned with the effectiveness of The Haven as a recovery tool from the perspective of service users and carers. Members aspired to embrace a critical consciousness regarding their condition and progress by entering into a creative dialogue with each other. This began to create a network of understanding in the Research Group, amongst research participants and within The Haven community as a whole where transcripts were made widely available with attendees' permission.

Each person seemed to see their involvement in a different way ranging from the disinterested, the interested on-looker, the keen participant in the service evaluation process and focus groups, to a committed co-researcher with major involvement in the collaborative process of mapping the journey of recovery in personality disorder. Each client was free to participate in the way that they wished.

Numerical and other informal data was also collected. Since its inception, a broad range of numerical data had been recorded and statistically presented at The Haven for all clients. This data was collected for monitoring purposes for the Department of Health and local Commissioners and had also been required as part of a National Evaluation of the 11 Personality Disorder Pilot Projects. At The Haven this data encompassed 166 clients by the end of the study and included number registered, gender, age, ethnicity, reason for referral, and outcomes about the use of the wider service area before and after registering at The Haven. Some of this information has been used as background data to enrich the study by augmenting the analysis of themes numerically. All service users at The Haven were invited to participate in the user-led Haven Community Advisory Group Meetings and Community Discussions. Here the dialogue was augmented and continued on a day-to-day, month-to-month basis. All meetings were minuted and relevant contents were also used as background data to illustrate themes.

Who took part?

Known as *sampling*, in qualitative research studies the aim is to provide an in-depth examination of meaning and its diversity. Parker (1994) considers that a qualitative researcher should state very clearly why a particular selection of participants was made, and highlights the moral responsibility placed on the researcher in relation to convenience and volunteer sampling, which involves a selection of the most accessible and willing. He also highlights that the types of people who choose to take part in a study may be different, for example, brighter or friendlier. Although self-selected samples are justifiable in qualitative research, additional strategies are possible, such as purposive or judgemental sampling (Marshall 1996). Here researchers actively select what is considered to be the most productive sample in terms of specific experiences. Age, gender or social class may be important for a particular study. Consideration can also be given to negative case analysis (Henwood and Pidgeon 1994), that is, in order to address the self-selected nature of some of the sample, and questions regarding trustworthiness in the use of purposive or judgemental sampling, the selection of some participants for interview who disagree and who might have a disconfirming potential may be of value in assuring that any assumptions are sufficiently challenged. By making sure not to include only those people who would say good things, the aim was to capture a diversity of potential opinions.

The potential sample population at The Haven consisted of all those who had registered at the project, which totalled 166 by the end of the study. The overall number of participants involved in the formal data collection of the study was 60 clients and six carers. Self-selection from The Haven population sample was achieved by posters and mailings about the research and the ready availability of information sheets and consent forms at the service which opened up attendance at focus groups and individual interviews to all registered clients. This became what is known as convenience sampling which was expressed as self-selection and volunteering in attendance at various research meetings and interviews. The Research Group addressed this issue by also considering a degree of purposive and theoretical sampling. Here, consideration was given to age, gender, domiciliary situation, marital status, parenthood, education, and presenting problems. Two clients who had left The Haven in unsatisfactory circumstances, due to unacceptable behaviour issues, were also interviewed individually in order to test and challenge theories. Others were invited because of their comprehensive use of various parts of the service or because of marked positive change in terms of coping strategies. Table 4.1 on the following page shows the length of time each client participant had been registered at The Haven, how many research events each participant attended and the length of time each participant was involved in the study.

Table 4.1 The involvement of research participants

Length of time at The Haven	
Timescale	**Number of clients**
Under 6 months	3
6 months to 1 year	4
1 year to 2 years	12
2 years to 3 years	17
3 years to 3½ years	24
Total	**60**
Attendance at research events	
Event	**Number of clients**
1 event	24
2 events	20
3 events	5
4 events	1
5 events	2
6 events	3
7 events	1
8 events	2
10 events	1
11 events	1
Total	**60**
Time involved in the study	
Timescale	**Number of clients**
1 month	24
Up to 3 months	13
Up to 6 months	5
1 to 2 years	12
2 to 2¾ years	6
Total	**60**

Ethical issues

The research study met the criteria for ethical permission from the University Ethics Committee. Participants were asked in advance if they would like to take part in the study. They were provided with a comprehensive and comprehensible information sheet and signed a consent form to give informed consent and the option to withdraw at any stage. Confidentiality was protected by the use of pseudonyms and further assured by making certain that other identity indicators were amended in transcripts. Copies of verbatim transcripts were sent to all participants, giving them the opportunity to correct or further amend their contribution, should they wish, which some did. As described earlier, a service user researcher was trained and supported to facilitate focus groups and to carry out individual interviews and a carer was trained and supported to facilitate carer focus groups. This was to ensure that participants were not unduly influenced in their responses by being questioned by me, because I held the dual role of initiating researcher and Haven Chief Executive. However, I was present throughout all focus groups as an observer. This did not appear to have been inhibiting in terms of affecting the openness of responses from participants, nor in influencing their willingness to disagree or express criticisms. In fact, they seemed to react well to the presence of the Chief Executive, seeing it as an acknowledgement of the importance and value of their responses.

As mentioned earlier, facilitators were remunerated by receiving payment for conducting focus groups or individual interviews. Participants were also valued by being paid for the time they devoted to any attendance at a SEG, focus group or individual interview. Immediate support was provided should any participant become unduly distressed by attendance at a focus group or interview. This happened at research events on two occasions. First, a participant whose child had been taken into care became distressed when a discussion occurred about hopes and dreams of having children. Second, another participant became distressed while trying to define recovery as it seemed impossible to attain. Both participants received immediate support from Haven staff and the second returned to the focus group to continue the discussion.

A primary ethical issue is the importance of ensuring that the research findings will be of benefit to people. Participants should also not be misled about the true nature of the study (Robson 1997). Tindall (1994) discusses the importance of equalizing the power relationship and democratizing the process. This may be aided by promoting ownership of the research, and ensuring participants receive copies of interviews and transcripts, in order to generate shared understanding and an opportunity to view data objectively. Accountability in the research process begins with the purpose of the study. What function does it serve and who is it for? Qualitative researchers make visible people's lives and can bring about social change. Who is to change, who decides the direction and who is authorized to recognize whether change has taken place? Who is the expert? Accountability, in all its facets, is an integral ethical issue, but it is often overlooked (Burman 1994). In addressing ethical issues regarding power and power-sharing, Tindall (1994) suggests that consciousness-raising in research often involves a one-way movement towards the researcher's understanding. However, in emancipatory research, when change occurs the role of the researcher as agent for change is less central and powerful than the group as a whole (Beresford and Wallcraft 1997; Winter and Munn-Giddings 2001). The Research Diary throughout, Appendix II, reflects the collaborative nature of the study, from the discussion of concepts, the creation of research questions, the scheduling and carrying out of data collection, to the data analysis.

Data analysis

The data collection process spanned two and three-quarter years. By March 2007 we had already amassed approximately 600 pages of verbatim transcripts. By the end of data collection, in November 2007, this amounted to 770 pages. Data analysis took one and a half years. During the data collection phase of the study challenges to the timescale had occurred from the outset in terms of the sheer volume of work involved in setting up a new service. Staffing difficulties had also caused delays and the cancellation of Research Group meetings for several months in 2006. I questioned the possibility of being able to continue the study. Members of the Research Group were determined it should continue and staff offered extra service support to enable this to happen. During the data analysis phase, after all we had experienced prior to this time, the fact that I had sustained a mere broken wrist did not seem at all to be a significant barrier to continuing the analysis. Unfortunately it was my right wrist, but I mastered the art of one-handed typing. Within the context of my time-limited study schedule, the year and a half taken to analyze the data was mainly attributable to its great volume and to the testing of methods by which the findings could be effectively evaluated.

It was crucial to us that I should not carry out this analysis alone. In the spirit of participatory research the Research Group would be involved every step of the way. In analyzing the research we chose to use *thematic analysis* as our method. This is a systematic way of searching for themes amongst a large quantity of data. It is carried out by coding the data, descriptively and interpretively, in order to reveal those themes (Braun and Clarke 2006). Here, data from focus groups and interviews could be classified and related, into themes, ideas and theories. Data from service evaluation groups, community discussions, and advisory meetings further augmented the study by being similarly coded and analyzed for related themes.

All theoretical frameworks carry a number of assumptions about the data and a good thematic analysis makes this transparent. Therefore, following is a detailed description of our analysis. Whittaker (2009) presents a six-stage approach in a graphic and palatable way, as follows:

1. *Becoming familiar with the data* necessitates an immersion in the material involving repeated reading in order to search for patterns and meaning. Although it can be time consuming and it may be tempting to skip over this stage, this is not advisable as it is the bedrock of the analysis. A familiarity with our data already existed. Transcripts had been circulated, read and re-read. I had been present at every focus group. Our participant researcher, who had facilitated research events, had been present at every focus group and interview. At the Research Group meeting in March 2007, the group had already begun to list ideas for themes emerging from the data. During December 2007 I read through all data again, manually marking some of the major themes with coloured pens. Here, I began to mark areas for coding which would develop throughout the entire analysis. This required very detailed reading of individual interviews and focus groups together with service evaluation group transcripts and minutes of client meetings at The Haven.

2. *Creating initial codes* began after the familiarization with the data produced a list of ideas about what was relevant in the research material. In this phase the initial coding of the data was organized into groups that could be related to themes. Fuller and Petch (1995) suggest that confronting a pile of raw data can be a daunting prospect and that analysis with the help of a computer software package for social sciences can greatly aid the process. The quantity of data in our study benefited from the use of the Nvivo7 computer software package. With the use of Nvivo7 I coded the

transcripts into 14 categories, or nodes, and these are listed in Research Group meeting minutes of January 2008 (Appendix II). This coding of data differed from the analysis of themes, which was broader. For example, the Research Group produced a list of initial ideas about themes relating to recovery in the March 2007 Research Group meeting which began with the need to feel safe. However, as transcripts were more closely examined, related sub-categories emerged which included for example, the importance of being welcomed, of kindness and being listened to.

3. *Searching for themes* begins when all the data has been initially coded and compiled into a list. These themes were worked on by assigning transcripts to different Research Group members at our Research Group meeting in January 2008. From January to August 2008 we worked on the 14 transcripts. During this time, with the use of Nvivo7, I also constructed 60 additional nodes by creating individual transcripts for each client participant. This was done with the idea of including some individual case studies in the research report. Unified themes began to emerge during the Research Group's work on the analysis as we refocused at the broader level of themes and began to analyze the codes and to consider how they might combine into a unified theme. Here, for example, we began to see that issues of safety, and the importance of matters such as being listened to, seemed to constitute a broad primary category about safety and trust.

4. *Reviewing themes* occurs once a set of initially qualifying themes has been devised. Themes are refined by discarding those with insufficient data to support them, or if the data is too diverse. Two themes might form one and other themes may need to be broken down into more than one. If the thematic map works then the researcher should move on to the next phase, if not, further review and refining of codes should occur. By this time, as well as the electronically themed nodes, we had an additional pile of handwritten analyses of these transcripts which had been produced by the efforts of the Research Group. These related the aspects of the various nodes to each other and suggested broader themes. The 60 individual node transcripts also showed clear patterns of improvement for individual clients over time.

However, at our Research Group meeting in August 2008, I spoke to members about my growing realization that we had missed out a step in our analysis and that I felt a further refining of data was needed. At the beginning of the data analysis I had considered organizing responses to each research question, numerically into themes. This step had been omitted, not just because 66 participants were involved, but also because many clients had answered the same question more than once. Some had answered questions multiple times at different research events. The

SEG questions had also changed in sequence over time and had become refined into focus group questions. The individual interview questionnaire contained additional questions. The carer focus group questions also included differences. In terms of timescale, this represented a great deal of complex work.

The Research Group agreed that it was very important to see the breakdown of responses to questions in terms of their themes and also their incidences. Three months was the target set for me to conduct this breakdown of findings from each individual research question. I felt it was important to stress to the Research Group that their work on the thematic analysis had not been wasted. In fact, it was crucial that all parts of the findings and analyses eventually worked in unison to produce themes that would fit together in a way that would tell a story about our data. From September 2008 to January 2009 transcripts of the findings from the research questions were distributed to members of the Research Group for comment. By the end of January 2009 the analysis of findings from the questions was complete. University research supervisors considered these findings were too lengthy to incorporate into the research report. However, they have been included in this book as Appendix VII: Findings from Clients' Questions, and Appendix VIII: Findings from Family and Carer Questions. Removing the findings, which had stemmed from the questions, into the appendices enabled us to focus on the primary research topic of recovery for people with personality disorder. The next stage of the analysis, described below, represented a meta-analysis of all the data collected during the study.

5. *Defining and naming themes* required a further analysis of the data within them. A write-up of each theme needed to occur, outlining what it was about, what was of interest and why and how it fitted into the overall story. Now it was possible to continue the thematic analysis with further coding carried out on all transcripts. A variety of nodes was compiled and compared as a verification of data within transcripts. This offered opportunities for reflection, enabling a rich analysis of themes against some of the numerical incidences of their occurrence. At the Research Group meeting in March 2009 I presented the analysis of the first two themes to members and we spoke about the third proposed theme. A further discussion occurred about later themes. At the May 2009 meeting I circulated the transcript for the first four themes and, fundamentally informed by the service user members of the Research Group, an in-depth discussion occurred about later themes and how the first four related to them. By June 2009 the first draft of the thematic analysis had been sent to the 66 research respondents. I had presented themes in the journey of recovery for personality disorder

graphically, as a Maslow-type pyramid (1943), and the Research Group liked this because they felt it represented growth and progress.

6. *Producing the report* should tell the complex story of the data in a way which convinces the reader of its value and the thoroughness of the analysis. Therefore, the report needed to provide more than just data. It needed to be convincing and compelling in a way that used narrative to illustrate our story. The findings are presented in the next chapter, Chapter 5, first as a series of tables providing background data, then as a profiling of the sample against the overall Haven population, and as an outlining of some of the domiciliary and life circumstances of participants. Numerical analyses of service cost-savings are also presented. Finally, consideration is given to each theme in the journey of recovery in personality disorder. As already explained, the findings from the research questions are included as Appendices VII and VIII. Within these appendices efforts were made to include quotations from all participants, ensuring their voices were uniformly heard. Selected quotations have been liberally included in the next chapters because we felt it was important that the story was told, as far as possible, in participants' words. Although we had planned to include some case studies in the research report there was insufficient space to do so. More recent case studies do, however, form the basis of Chapter 8, which is the penultimate chapter of this book.

One theme that only I worked on concerned organizational learning and change. Although I analyzed this data against Haven records, to ensure fidelity of timescale regarding organizational changes, the Research Group continued to comment on emerging data and the results as they were written up. This is included as Chapter 7 and, consistent with our action research approach, it shows the way in which emerging data from the research was used to effect change and growth within The Haven.

CHAPTER 5

Discoveries on the Journey of Recovery

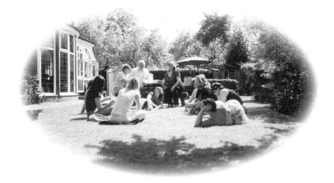

Before I came to The Haven I used to overdose on a reasonably regular basis, I used to cut myself whenever anything went wrong, and I used to stop eating when anything went wrong. Basically it was a whole host of maladaptive coping mechanisms and, since coming to The Haven, I have sort of redressed these. The difference is now I can rationalize the situation enough to think what would be the actual impact of doing it. It's the actual stopping and analyzing the situation for what it really is, not what emotionally it's built itself up to be.

Service User Quotation

Before describing our discoveries, our core findings on the journey, a variety of background data is given to enrich the study by augmenting the analysis of themes numerically.

Background information and demographics ───────

Following are a number of tables which will help to further illustrate our discoveries by profiling The Haven population and the research participants. This data encompasses numbers registered at the service, sources of and reasons for referral, gender, age and ethnicity. Some of this data has been compared, numerically, with the research sample of participants. Additional information about the life circumstances of the research sample has been included, as have findings regarding the research participants' reduction in the use of psychiatric services during the course of the study.

Out of 166 Haven clients 60 clients were involved in this research study. Table 5.1 illustrates the overall Haven population; how many were using mental health services at the time they registered at The Haven; the source of referral for each and the reason for referral. These were the presenting problems for clients and most clients fell into more than one category.

Table 5.1 The Haven population

Haven clients	
Clients	**Number**
Total number of clients registered by the end of the study	166
Engaged with Mental Health Services at time of registration	144
Source of referral	
Source	**Number**
Self	45
Hospital/psychiatrist	41
Community Mental Health Team	33
GP	9
Other	8
Family and friends	7
Mind	7
Crisis Resolution and Home Treatment Team	5

Criminal Justice Mental Health Team	3
Housing providers	3
Assertive outreach	3
Psychology Department	2
Total	**166**
Reason for referral	
In many cases more than one presenting problem	**Number**
Severe depression/anxiety	139
Suicidal impulses	69
Self-harm	59
Substance misuse	45
Anti-social/violence/aggression	34
Isolation/inter-personal problems	30
Volatile moods/mood swings	28
Paranoia/voices	23
Eating disorder	18
Institutionalized long hospitalization/prison	6
Manic episodes	6
Obsessive-compulsive	4
Gender dysphoria/gender issues	3

In Table 5.2 on the following page the age range of The Haven population is shown and compared with the age range of research participants; gender for the overall Haven population compared with gender for research participants is shown; and ethnic origin of the overall Haven population compared to that of the research sample. This table reveals inclusion in the research study of a fairly representative cross section of participants, in terms of age, gender and ethnic origin, compared to the overall Haven population.

Table 5.2 Haven population compared to research participants

Age				
Age range	Overall clients	Percentage	Research clients	Percentage
18–20	5	3%	1	1.7%
21–24	9	5.4%	2	3.3%
25–34	41	24.7%	11	18.3%
35–44	66	39.8%	24	40%
45–54	34	20.5%	16	26.7%
55–65	11	6.6%	6	10%
Total	166	100%	60	100%
Gender				
Gender	Overall clients	Percentage	Research clients	Percentage
Male	43	25.9%	13	21.7%
Female	123	74.1%	47	78.3%
Total	166	100%	60	100%
Ethnicity				
Ethnic origin	Overall clients	Percentage	Research clients	Percentage
White British	156	94%	57	95%
British-born Pakistani	2	1.2%	1	1.7%
Irish	2	1.2%	0	0%
Irish/English	1	0.6%	0	0%
Dutch	1	0.6%	1	1.7%
German-born Romany gipsy	1	0.6%	0	0%
Mixed race white/Afro Caribbean	1	0.6%	0	0%
Mixed race white/Asian Indian	1	0.6%	0	0%

White American – USA	1	0.6%	1	1.7%
Total	**166**	**100%**	**60**	**100%**

Table 5.3 illustrates some of the history of the research sample in relation to whether they were in care as children; had a forensic history; had ever been employed; or were in employment at the time they registered at The Haven. It also shows domiciliary situation, and relationships in terms of whether research participants were single, or separated, in a relationship, if they had children and whether they retained care of their children. This table also shows the sample's use of statutory mental health services by the end of the study and reveals that hospital admissions for research participants during the last year of the study had dropped to seven. Finally, it shows that more than half of the research sample was completely discharged from mental health services by the end of the study.

Table 5.3 Further profiling of the research participants

Some life circumstance					
Life circumstances	**Male Yes**	**Female Yes**	**Total Yes**	**Total No**	**Total**
Been in care	4	17	21	39	60
Forensic history	10	9	19	41	60
Ever been employed	9	23	32	28	60
In employment when came to The Haven	0	2	2	58	60
Accommodation					
Type			**Number**		
Rented accommodation			41		
Owner occupier			12		
Supported accommodation			4		
Living with parents			3		
Total			**60**		

Relationships and children	
Situation	**Number**
Single and no children	23
In a relationship and children	10
Single and children	9
Single with children in care	8
In a relationship with children in care	6
In a relationship and no children	4
Total	**60**
In psychiatric hospital during the last year of the study	
	Number
No	53
Yes	7
Total	**60**
Discharge from statutory mental health services by end of study	
	Number
No	28
Yes	32
Total	**60**

Use of services and cost-savings

Additional background data which illustrates our findings concerns the use of other services. By 2006, an analysis of use of the wider service area for the first 50 Haven clients who had been with the project for one year, showed a drop in all services measured as shown in Table 5.4. Notably, psychiatric hospital in-patient admissions had dropped for the first 50 clients by 85 per cent. Although continuing to represent a burden for GPs and the A&E Department, use had still dropped by 25 per cent and 45 per cent respectively.

Calculating the reduction of the use of the wider service area, in Table 5.4, against health and social care figures, showed that the project had saved £220,000 over and above the cost of The Haven, for the first 50 clients alone. By this time we had registered 110 clients and extrapolating savings to that number showed that in excess of £480,000 could be saved, over and above the cost of running the service. The cost per week, per client for Haven services was around £100, compared to costs ranging from £223 to £1250 per patient per week for personality disorder day unit or hospital therapeutic community, in other parts of the country (Chiesa *et al.* 2002).

Table 5.4 The first 50 Haven clients to complete one year at The Haven

Service area/ intervention	Annual average use over two years prior to Haven	Annual service use since attending The Haven	Percentage reduction in use of service/ intervention
Section 136	42.5 times	18 times	57.64%
Other sections	11 times	4 times	63.63%
Psychiatric in-patient admissions	55 times	8 times	85.45%
Use of day hospital	32 clients	14 clients	56.25%
Use of community MH team	36 clients	14 clients	61.11%
Use of NERIL (MH Help-line)	1264 times	317 times	75.92%
Use of crisis team	187 times	42 times	77.54%
Criminal justice MH team	0	0	0
Assertive outreach	0	0	0
Trust eating disorder service	56 times	14 times	75.00%
Psychology/ psychotherapy/ counselling	30 clients	21 clients	30.00%
Annual use of GP	611 times	459 times	24.87%

Service area/ intervention	Annual average use over two years prior to Haven	Annual service use since attending The Haven	Percentage reduction in use of service/ intervention
Annual use of A&E	141 times	77 times	45.39%
General hospital admissions	47 times	37 times	21.27%
Police/probation/ prison	12.5 times	2 times	84.00%
Children's social services	14 clients	6 clients	57.14%
Debt agencies	7 clients	1 client	85.71%
Housing/ homelessness	11 clients	2 clients	81.81%
Substance misuse voluntary agency	4 clients	1 client	75.00%
Eating disorder voluntary agency	5 clients	1 client	80.00%
Mind advocate	39 clients	11 clients	71.79%

The Haven had, therefore, fulfilled its original promise to engage the client group in our area and to prove cost savings in the wider service area. However, concerns began to be expressed about whether the project would create a new kind of dependency. Although the National Personality Disorder Team had allowed us the latitude necessary to develop a pilot service, during 2006 it was local Commissioners who had begun to mention words like 'through-put' and 'discharge'. They questioned our ability to address capacity at the service if this through-put did not occur. Many clients had complex needs and long psychiatric histories. We knew that we had some clients who had gone from adolescent sexual abuse to adolescent psychiatric treatment units and then to adult psychiatric secure units for a decade or more. One client came to us after 36 years in special hospitals and secure units. The treatment time-scale envisaged by local Commissioners was highly unrealistic. Most of the 110 clients who had registered were still with us and, although many were no longer subject to hospital admission, questions were asked about whether they could move beyond the stability achieved at The Haven. These questions did indeed have a bearing on capacity at the project and the need to continue to register new clients. Therefore, in response to these concerns and as a result of emerging findings of this study, The Haven developed a new way of working with capacity and opened a social inclusion unit at the service. This organizational change is described in Chapter 7.

Before leaving the subject of wider service use and cost-savings, it is worth noting that The North Essex Mental Health NHS Trust updated the service savings analysis in 2009, suggesting that the average annual reduction in the use of their services had been maintained over a four year period as shown in Table 5.5.

Table 5.5 Mental Health Trust analysis of service use 2005 to 2009 (Date Source: Care Base Date 22 June 2009)

Service	Two year average before Haven	Four year average after Haven
Number of inpatient spells	111	*
Number of Section 136s	*	*
Number of other sections	*	*
Number of attendances in day care services	2364	177
Number of attendances in outpatient services	370	39
Number of attendances in CMHT services (Community MH Team)	1196	124
Number of attendances in CRHT services (Crisis Resolution & Home Treatment)	168	*
Number of attendances in CJMHT services (Criminal Justice MH Team)	*	*

Service	Two year average before Haven	Four year average after Haven
Number of attendances in AO services (Assertive Outreach)	71	*
Number of attendances in substance misuse services	*	*
Number of attendances in eating disorder/ nutritional advisor services	169	*
Number of attendances psychology/ psychological/counselling services	287	*
Number of attendances in other services	*	*

* Any breakdown of data where the aggregated numbers are less than 30, are not reported due to patient confidentiality.

It is also important to emphasize that The Haven repeated this exercise in 2013, with the last 50 clients registered at the project, and the significant reduction in the use of the wider service area, after one year at The Haven, continued to be maintained. A chart combining the analyses for 2006 and 2013 has been included as Appendix IX.

Findings from the questions to research participants

As outlined in Chapter 4, because of the vast amount of data collected at research events during the course of the study, findings from the research questions have been compiled into appendices. Here, data from the 34 research events has been categorized against the questions asked. Responses to each question have been further broken down into categories or themes suggested by the responses. These have been listed numerically in descending order from highest to lowest. Appendix VII shows the *Findings from Client Questions* and Appendix VIII shows the *Findings from Family and Carer Questions*. Pseudonyms chosen by participants, to protect identity, are consistent throughout the data in the appendices and chapters.

Mapping the process of recovery

Findings from the groups and interviews, in the research transcripts and in Appendices VII and VIII, together with all data collected during the study, has been subject to the thematic analysis described in the last chapter. An examination of emerging themes within and between transcripts and questions, and the interplay between themes, gives insight into what the participants considered to be the key steps in the journey of recovery for someone with a personality disorder diagnosis. Themes are initially presented diagrammatically as a pyramid representing a hierarchy of progress (Figure 5.1).

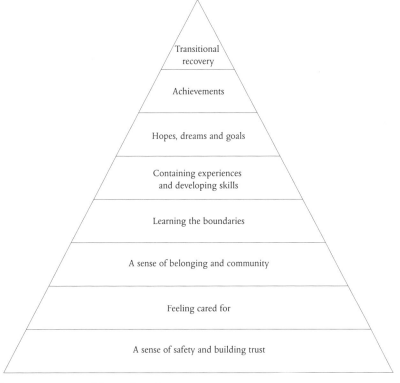

Figure 5.1 Haven hierarchy of progress:
The journey of recovery for personality disorder.

The themes are now considered, each in turn, and are illustrated by data extracts in the form of participant quotations. Although many participants have said similar things about particular themes, the quotations have been selected here because of their particular expressiveness.

A sense of safety and building trust

Whatever we might call the difficulties experienced by those who had attracted a diagnosis of personality disorder, be it disrupted attachment experiences or unresolved trauma, they came to The Haven robbed of central aspects of identity, memory, and feelings, sometimes resulting in widely swinging emotions, chronic hyper-arousal, terror, rage, despair, hopelessness, guilt and shame. Thoughts were sometimes incomprehensible and overwhelming and the need for physical and psychological *safety* was palpable. The first lesson in our study was that respondents were able to define the component parts of a *safe* place:

Igor: You can feel it when you walk in that door, you can feel that safety. It's a safe place. It helps you to be safe.

Crystal: I think The Haven is my place of safety, I feel relaxed.

Phoenix: It's probably the first time in my life I've felt safe enough to be in a group and taking part without constantly looking over my shoulder.

Participants explained that feeling safe related to an increased ability to protect them from the harm they might do to themselves:

Katy: Sometimes, just what I need at night time is to come in and know I'm safe and it stops me from doing anything at the moment.

Harry: The Haven's my safe space when I get really panicky and instead of running off in my car and ending up in the middle of nowhere, I'm more likely to come here now, which actually helps my family a lot because they are not so stressed because they know I am somewhere safe.

New clients at The Haven also identified, at an early stage, that a sense of safety was an important factor in preventing harm:

Roosle: I'm new to The Haven so I'm just learning what it can do right now. I'm using it as a safe place from myself, because I'm in a very dangerous and unsafe state and it's a place where I can go where I know I won't come to any harm.

Additionally, family members highlighted safety as an important element:

Alex: I feel, definitely, it's helped my daughter. It's somewhere safe for her to come, somewhere without any bad memories.

Sarah: I knew that I could probably go to sleep and that he was going to be okay and safe.

Participants also identified that responsiveness engendered a sense of safety, enabling feelings to be expressed and *trust* to be built. Responsiveness was cited both in terms of the vital necessity of 24-hour service availability and as emotional responsiveness:

May: It makes me feel very safe and secure to know it's always there. To me it's safe 24/7, it's a haven. That's what it really means.

Abigail: Its all-round 24-hour support is something that I've really found helpful, knowing that there's someone there. It gives you a sort of safety net.

Gemma: I came in here on Monday and burst into tears, and I hadn't done that for some time beforehand, and a member of staff took me into the Safe Centre and she said, 'You're here now, you're safe, you can let your feelings go, cry all you want, you don't have to pretend anymore,' and that was such lovely words to hear that I didn't have to wear this mask or put on a smile or brave face.

Participants also described the helpfulness of a consistent approach in relation to trust and safety:

Brunhilda: I've been very upset and, each time I've spoken to a staff member, I haven't had to go through the same story each time, they all seem to know what's happening with me, so it's very helpful.

May: I think that the way things are handed over, when you are in crisis you don't have to tell your story all over again from the beginning, because the people you speak to on the phone, or in a one-to-one, know enough about your symptoms and situation, and that makes it much easier.

Conversely, responses showed that trust can be easily shattered if someone is let down by a lack of availability, consistency or responsiveness. In relation to organizational learning and change, Chapter 7 describes that adjustments in the telephone crisis service were made because of participant responses:

Chloe:　But, if you're seeing someone in a one-to-one you can't have them constantly jumping up to answer the phone because it just doesn't work, you know, like there's no continuity. You're made to feel unimportant and the phone takes priority and that's not good enough.

Carers and family members also highlighted the crucial importance of building trust:

Alex:　You've gained the trust I think, which is one of the things when people come out of hospital, or before they come here, that they haven't got trust in anything. I mean the people that love and care for them, not in the mental health system, they don't trust anyone. But when they come here it's a gradual trust in people. They don't feel they are going to be let down and that's a big positive and then they gradually can begin even to trust themselves to do things and take responsibility.

The degree of trust experienced, in relation to past services, was described by participants:

Tom:　It's a lot to do with trust though isn't it? I trust, completely, I trust every one of you. Whereas, with the other places, it's phew, there's no trust there. They let you down and it's gone.

Participants described how feeling safe and learning to trust enabled them to stop hiding their emotions and to begin to explore their feelings and experiences:

Igor:　For me The Haven has taught me to trust again and respect other people. It's through this place that I've learned I don't have to hide my problems; I don't have to hide behind a smile anymore. I can come in and cry, I can be me for once. I think the important thing really is that coming here makes you safe enough to change.

Feeling cared for

Participants also revealed the importance of *feeling cared for* as a finding and described a component of *care* in terms of first contact and acceptance; acceptance no matter what:

Phoenix: They always look pleased to see you coming through the door.

Daniel: Every time I've come here everyone has made me feel really welcome.

Fred: I've phoned when I've been in crisis and I've always been welcomed no matter what my mood or what's going through my head.

Participants knew about the affection that can exude from a smile and the warmth than can be felt from a hug or simply being made a cup of tea:

Doris: It's been excellent, a kind ear, a cuddle, cup of tea, respite when I need it.

Chloe: I don't do hugs, but I do now.

Norris: It's the sort of place you can get a hug or give one. When I first came here I couldn't let anyone near me, or in my space, without being completely drunk, this was outside here, and now I can. Most of the time people can hug me and be close to me without, you know, that would have never happened before I started coming here, without me being under the influence.

They spoke of being listened to and treated as if they were important:

Gemma: The calmness, softness of the staff they make you feel… they make you a cup of tea or coffee and they listen, they listen. They let you talk, they let you speak, they let you cry and they hand you tissues. You know I never…care and genuine care, absolutely wonderful.

Brunhilda: One of the most important things is the human-ness of The Haven staff and other clients, there's a kind of warmth and compassion.

Charles: There are people who give a shit, you know.

85

Family members and carers concurred regarding the importance of the warm, friendly and caring response at The Haven:

Sarah: To be honest I found the hospital a hustle and bustle. I don't really think I got any help at all. I can honestly say I got nowhere, absolutely nowhere. I have to say, I might have a tear in a minute, I have to say that The Haven is just, it's a wonderful place really. I really mean that.

Participants highlighted the touch of pampering and complementary therapies, and of interconnectedness and humanness:

Chloe: The only time I'm really touched is when I come here, because I live by myself and don't have a partner. Somebody actually touching you makes you feel that you are valuable as a person. Touch is really important.

Kim: I love the face packs, or my hands being done, I feel like a queen.

Participants also spoke about how feeling cared for made one feel special and valued and how this had contributed to beginning to feel better about oneself:

Rose: I think they make you feel special and that's quite a hard thing to do.

Tiffany: The staff try their hardest to make you feel very special in your own individual way, and they give you loads of boosts of confidence you know.

Doris: You are important. The staff treat us as humans, so we think we are human, rather than part of a different species. Since coming to The Haven I got to a period where I thought, yeah I do like myself a bit more.

A sense of belonging and community

Our families are supposed to provide a place in which we feel safe and learn to trust, where we feel cared for and where we develop and learn to be spontaneous and creative. Clients at The Haven had often found this not to be the case and they came to us instead with a legacy of abuse, neglect, abandonment or a lack of emotional responsiveness. The next finding to emerge from the study was about the sense of belonging that the community generated. This was experienced as a reciprocal relationship where common ground was identified; you are broken like me:

Carl: I find when you walk into the room the thing I like about all of them is everybody has got the same illness, same problems, and this is where The Haven comes into its own, because they recognize those problems, and they are able to help you.

Emily: I isolate and can't mix with people, but I can see people in The Haven, you are the same as me.

Participants expressed how this had led to a sense of belonging and fitting in, perhaps for the first time:

Lara: It's taken a long time, but I finally feel that this is the place where I fit in and I feel comfortable, I feel comfortable around the people here, it's very nice.

Anne: One of my hopes, dreams was to fit in, into this world, and being at The Haven I think I've finally started to fit in.

Family members and carers also pinpointed the importance of The Haven as a specialist community:

Sammy: The Haven serves a specialist community in a very specialist way. The hospitals and the community mental health teams, their only specialty is mental health, where The Haven is catering for a group of people and a limited number so, actually, you can work far better with those individuals and be more focused, so we certainly don't want it to go away.

Rob: I think that's the definition of a community as opposed to a service.

Participants voiced a clear awareness and understanding that they were part of a community and that this was very different from other services they had experienced:

Rose: I haven't seen any NHS mental health people run things like this.

Jenny: I don't think I've ever been any place where there have been people around me that have got mental health problems and there's been such a good strength of community.

David: Without the community spirit that's here I think a lot of people would be in hospital, or even worse than that, if it wasn't for the people here.

Decision-making was shared, bonds of friendship were made. There was fun:

Gemma: There's always people around and you can hear them laughing, precious company.

Chloe: I haven't laughed as much in years at the last Friendship Group I came to here. It was just hilarious.

Anne: It's what The Haven is all about; it's being there for each other through good times and bad.

Negative aspects of community were also expressed by some, initially as a sense of alienation engendered by seeing others making friendships and joining in:

Sheila: I see everyone interacting with each other and caring for each other, and everything, and I'm sort of on the sidelines wishing I could join in and not able to.

Phoenix: I struggle with this idea of community. Sometimes I feel very, very threatened, and sometimes I feel very safe, sometimes I feel comforted, but there are times I feel threatened and vulnerable.

Participants expressed satisfaction in the community working and striving together for common goals:

Brunhilda: It's such a great representation of what you would call a community, and I personally have looked for a community for several years, and this is really what I think community ought to be because it's staff and clients all together have created this place.

Ultimately, many participants, including family members and carers, identified that a central component to this theme was that The Haven community had given members a sense of home and family:

Pablo: The Haven provides for me a replacement role of my parental home.

Ben: It feels that you are a replacement Mum and Dad that I never had.

Alex: She's got friends here, I think she feels even the staff are her friends as well, and I just feel that she feels that is more of her home now. This has taken the place of her home.

May: It's the family I never had.

Learning the boundaries

The next finding concerned the limits of acceptable behaviour. If The Haven is likened to an exercise in re-parenting, in addition to nurturing and love, this needed to include firm *boundaries* which imposed limits on unacceptable behaviour. The findings revealed that boundaries needed to be known and democratically negotiated and administered:

Boris: I suppose the biggest issue for me would have to be the boundaries of The Haven, and the policies need to be kept because to aid someone's recovery you need boundaries and that's what so many people lack.

Doris: We all do things that are socially unacceptable but it is really better to make them a little less acceptable, like they are in the big wide world.

This theme emerged as a potential lesson, or barrier, on the journey of recovery. This was discussed by the Research Group at their meeting in May 2009, Appendix II, as the first four themes began to emerge. In this part of the data analysis Haven polices and minutes of client meetings were included and used to augment data collected from focus groups and interviews.

The Haven's Acceptable Behaviour Policy was created in collaboration with its clients and administered by the clients. If a Haven community member broke the rules laid out in this policy there were consequences, and that client would be invited to a community discussion with peers if a boundary had been clearly transgressed. Minutes were kept for community discussions and sent out to all Haven clients. During the first year of operation at The Haven, research participants began to discuss behavioural issues at community discussion meetings, as follows. The issue under discussion below concerned a client in a crisis/respite bed at the project who had self-harmed:

Jonny: It made me feel so upset that I felt like not coming to The Haven again. Although I do want to stress that I know this person is very unwell, really suffering and in need of help.

Abigail: I have struggled against unacceptable behaviours because a crisis bed is a privilege and, if someone breaks the rules, there are usually many others trying to keep the rules who need the bed.

Alexis: What if someone breaks the rules by, for example, self-harming in their sleep?

This latter query was answered by staff, 'You tell me, you are the ones making the rules.' The conclusion from this early discussion was that a stay in a bed should be terminated if a client self-harmed. Other bed stays would be booked in the future for this client, but further similar occurrences from any client should be acted on immediately, as above, thereby providing a clear boundary and consistency of approach.

Community discussions during our second year of operation included alcohol issues, resulting in a several week ban for one client, for which this was a second offence, and who had caused serious upset and disruption in the project and outside in the car park. On return to the project at the end of the ban the client requested a further community discussion and made the following statement:

Calvin: All clients here have issues and one of them is alcohol for quite a few people. The last thing you need is for someone to turn up under the influence of alcohol. I sincerely apologize and I'm really sorry for all the upset I caused.

Further observations from research participants clearly revealed that in order to be effective a boundary should be stronger than the impulse to engage in dysfunctional actions. This became a deterrent explicit in the rules, which could bar access to the project if the boundary was broken. In order to be strong enough the boundary needed to potentially take something away if it was broken, something greatly desired like a crisis bed or access to the project. Here a research participant reflected on this lesson learned regarding acceptable behaviour and alcohol:

Karen: About my bed, unfortunately, through my own stupid fault I consumed alcohol on my fifth day and had to go home. I was excluded for six days, but was offered telephone support and then I could come back after six days. A bed here I think is a great privilege and I have been told that I can have a second chance which I am extremely very, very grateful for, because it was a very stupid thing to do. I shall never lose my bed again. I've learnt my lesson.

Issues of drug misuse were also brought to the community for discussion. On one occasion it was discovered that a client had brought cannabis to the project while staying in a bed and had given it to two other clients. Strong feelings were expressed by both staff and clients regarding the fact that illegal drugs on site put the whole project at risk:

Brunhilda: Drugs are not the same as alcohol.

Leska: Closing the beds or police involvement would be punishing clients who are blameless.

The community decided to impose a four-week ban with telephone support and additionally a six-month veto on bed stays for this particular client. This discussion was also followed by the decision to institute an amnesty regarding all offences against the acceptable behaviour policy since the project's inception. This yielded a cathartic harvest of confessions which provided very interesting reading. The community agreed that, thereafter, any instances of illegal drugs on the premises, or any discussions or phone calls occurring at the premises about obtaining illegal drugs, would mean that the police were contacted immediately:

Wilf: It's brilliant that we run it, and we decide what happens. It's never nice to ban people and things like that, but at certain times we have to, you know, be stricter and I think that's starting to happen now, and I think, well since the amnesty, I think it has cleared the air, and I think we've become stronger now.

Discussions and learning about overdosing at the project usually proved more emotive, as clients examined and empathized with desperate emotional states which can precede this kind of behaviour. Although such occurrences were rare at The Haven, one client repeated this behaviour in just over a period of one year. The first instance prompted support and sympathy at the community discussion and the vote was in favour of no ban, but rather community service at the project in the form of work in the vegetable garden. The next occurrence, a year later, happened overnight while the same client was in a bed. After being taken to A&E and receiving the all-clear from the hospital the next day, the client returned to The Haven and excerpts from the subsequent community discussion are as follows. It is important to bear in mind that the client in question was present at the discussion and, although too upset to speak, heard all that was said:

Katy: It's very hard to discuss this kind of thing because we have all been there and can sympathize and understand.

Tiffany: I wonder why we have to punish someone for something like this.

Emily: We can all sympathize and empathize, but someone has to take responsibility for the consequences of their actions.

Crystal: Everyone will think they can do it. Thank goodness the person has not passed away. How would staff have felt if they had found them and how would clients have felt?

Daniel: If that had happened there would have been a Board of Enquiry and our funding could be taken away.

Doris: The person who has done this is a very dear friend and I love them to pieces, but we are all aware that when you feel like that you can go and talk to staff, and I'm not sure we can be too sympathetic as people will be cutting themselves and hanging from the pergola.

Boris: The decision we make today is very important and that's why we set the boundaries. We have got to keep the place safe and treat everyone exactly the same.

The community decided on a one-week ban, obviously with all necessary external support, and although the client left the meeting in tears, they have not to this day taken an overdose, either at The Haven or anywhere else.

In The Haven's later years, community discussions were well attended, with usually over 20 clients, seeing this function as part of their responsibility as community members. Some clients became seasoned in the process and quite skilled at, in the words of one client, 'tempering justice with mercy'. An example below concerns a client new to the project who displayed excessive attachment difficulties, refusing to leave the site on various occasions and even prompting staff to call the police for assistance, and who also overdosed en route to The Haven:

Brunhilda: We need to remember that this person is relatively new to the project and very young and that it can take quite a long time before someone truly understands how the community works and that it is a two way thing.

Doris: Many of us have been like this in the early days and demanded a whole heap of attention by reacting to boundaries. This person is still on a learning curve.

Boris: Would you like to have a buddy at the project, because I'm willing to act as your buddy?

In this instance the client was given a contract specifying points that needed to be adhered to, rather than a ban.

During research events, participants expressed a clear awareness of rules and a sense of safety and security about boundaries:

Sheila: I feel safe at The Haven because I know you're not allowed to get away with stuff, are you, like cutting while you're here, which means I don't try. It's about being protected from the negative parts of yourself.

Cosmic: I do get a real sense of freedom here, but I know that if anybody doesn't toe the line then they will be pulled up and they'll be at a meeting about it, yeah.

Further observations from research participants included learning about the impact one's behaviour has on others and taking back responsibility:

Jasmine: When I had my last stay here I actually self-harmed and got sent home. I took that very hard as a bed is like gold dust and I hated myself for doing that to the point where I was so scared to come back, but the staff kept persevering and managed to talk me round and I realized how much I was missing while I wasn't coming here. I used to use alcohol as a coping mechanism, and since The Haven I hardly drink alcohol anymore because if I've had a drink and I need to come in I won't be able to come in, so I make a real effort to keep off alcohol.

Jenny: It's good because you really get on with the staff so you actually respect them, you don't want to hurt them as well. You don't want them to feel bad. And it's not then just about you. You start to see that you are affecting other people as well. I think

93

that's the reason why they manage to sort us out a bit, because we actually like them all.

Pablo: It goes back to you taking your responsibility back really, that's what it's about. It's about giving you your responsibility back, not about losing responsibility.

Some family members and carers discussed the kinds of unacceptable behaviours that represented the burden of personality disorder, presenting severe stress for loved ones:

Rob: She tried to kill herself desperately under the care of the hospital and previous regimes.

Tony: She was stoned on Wednesday before her (family) turned up. I'm afraid that I'm at the end of my tether because of drugs and, as far as I'm concerned, are keeping her ill and she doesn't seem prepared to let it go. So, if you can help her in that aspect that might help. I'm also aware she's sold drugs, I'm really concerned. I caught her out at Christmas time drug dealing to children.

Sarah: At one stage, with my son, it was just like a rollercoaster, and I had family members saying to me, 'Just let him get on with it', you know, because my son would always ring me, and I would be going up to the hospital picking him up, or whatever, ambulances and all sorts, and I suppose as a Mum I couldn't not go.

Dinah: It's coping skills that we need and those are the strategies I hope The Haven will give to my partner. My partner has a ferocious temper and aggressive behaviours, and it's frightening, I find it very frightening, and for years I've put up with it, frightened in my own house, when she goes into one. We get these suicide attempts and we've been to hospital numerous times. I've run out of sympathy quite frankly because the first time it's, 'Oh my God', you know, the second times it's, 'Oh', the third time it's, 'Not again'. I'm not going to play the game anymore. I'm being pushed to a point that I'm having my strings pulled and I can't, I can't cope with all that manipulation that's being put on me.

94

Fifty-one clients, 85 per cent of participants, discussed the use of negative coping strategies during the course of the research and 46, over 76 per cent of participants, reported a reduction in their use, suggesting that the concept of boundaries had become internalized:

Pablo: My sobriety is unbelievable, my conscience is clear, I wake up clear. I mean the two things in my life that I do now that keep me together is that I eat well and I sleep well.

Leska: Since coming to The Haven I don't tie anything round my neck, I've had maybe one overdose and I've learned to talk and, when things get really bad, to phone and ask for support instead of acting on impulsive thoughts.

Alexis: I haven't touched alcohol for almost two years. I haven't self-harmed for almost 19/20 months with the help of The Haven's crisis line.

Fred: Taking drugs before, in the past, that was all I knew from the age of 13, what I'd learned in order to survive, basically, on the streets. I've come beyond that and my coping strategies are to talk I guess, and phone for help.

David: I'm not so aggressive as what I used to be like because I used to be a big bully.

Donald: I used to overdose probably once or twice a week and, in the last four or five months, that's stopped completely since I've come here. I never used to think about the consequences, I never used to think about who I was going to hurt, I never used to think there was other ways of dealing with things, and that you could actually talk to someone about things, instead of just doing it, so it's changed my life no end coming here.

Containing experiences and developing skills

The first four findings concerned developing healthy attachment in terms of safety and trust; feeling cared for; a sense of belonging; and learning acceptable boundaries, limits and behaviour. The next finding revealed that only when these were in place, and sufficiently consolidated, did respondents begin to learn to *contain* their past experiences and build necessary *skills* to progress. Meaningful therapy cannot take place, no matter how desperately it is needed, if trust does not exist and if behaviour is chaotic, risky and destructive. Healing is about integrating experience by making sense of what has happened. Prior to this stage, reality often proved to be unbearable and making sense out of traumatic experiences and child abuse is a difficult thing to do. This finding marked the long process of beginning to reframe traumatic experience.

In Figure 5.2, the pyramid of progress can be viewed in an alternative way, where the first four layers represent the foundations stones, or pillars, on which progress in the higher levels is built.

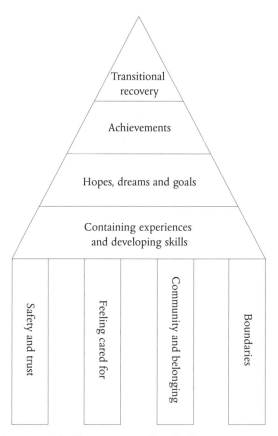

Figure 5.2 The pyramid of progress on foundation stones.

Prior to progress on the first four levels of the pyramid, difficulties had been experienced by many in simply being able to ask for help:

Sally: Sometimes you can see that staff are all busy, but you're too scared though, and you go home feeling worse, but it's too late. Then it's hard to pick up the phone.

Rose: Sometimes it is hard to pick up the phone so it is better that someone is phoning you.

When this began to change for participants, sometimes after a year or more of using the service, they began to develop, what to them were, the new skills of being able to ask for help and accept support:

Sally: I just used to sit in my flat and suffer in silence, but now I'm picking up the phone.

Rose: I am learning to actually ask for help before I act on things.

Participants indicated that their shift in the use of negative coping strategies was now intrinsically linked to asking for help rather than acting out:

Jenny: I used to self-harm a lot before I came here. Instead of doing that I've managed to pick up the phone. I used to like drink quite a lot as well, and knowing that if I do I can't come in here and speak to somebody, and I'd rather speak to somebody rather than pick up a drink.

In relation to feeling safe and building trust, participants had already spoken about beginning to let emotion out and about taking risks in talking about difficulties. Next came the process of beginning to analyze the experiences and emotions which were underlying feelings and behaviours:

Bling: I was having an adult conversation, as a normal 33-year-old would. All of a sudden something in my brain said, 'No that's not alright you effing cow, who do you think you are to judge me, well I'll see you in the effing hospital then when I've taken another overdose, bitch.' When I got angry it was how the 13-year-old child, how the teenager would deal with things, instead of what I'd call a normal adult, and it would be something like, 'Well I hope you die in a car crash on your way home,' until I got the help that I wanted.

Elise: I think my new skills have fundamentally been to be able to stop and question the reality of the situation and the most logical conclusions, and the most logical assumptions, and to think the whole situation through, rather than jump into the first panic stricken thought that comes into my head and act on it.

The statements above highlight changes in the use of negative coping strategies, and the ability to *contain experiences*. This ability had not emerged in this theme simply by learning the boundaries but also by reflection and realizations during therapeutic work in groups and individually. Participants spoke about building therapeutic skills in a variety of ways, for example, by learning to write about their emotions:

Anne: I am finding creative writing extremely helpful, it's helping me to get a lot of my emotions out on to paper and being able to share them with other people as well has always been hard for me, but I've started to read out my work.

Boris: Here I have broken the cycle of the pattern of behaviour into more constructive ways of dealing with it. Self-harming, or picking up a bottle of wine, I tend more now to put pen to paper and let it out that way.

Participants also spoke about learning skills in groups such as life skills and DBT (dialectical behaviour therapy) skills group:

Alexis: I feel I've really benefited from the life skills group; it's reduced my obsessional behaviour and encouraged me to mix with others and has really boosted my self-esteem. It's been very beneficial dealing with anxiety, positive thinking, how to control panic attacks, confidence building and particularly in dealing with anger.

Lara: I'm learning an awful lot in DBT, mindfulness, thinking before you speak, trying to change your actions and the way you think. I used to go off the handle at anything, now I stop to think of a different way of coping with it and a different way of speaking to people and it's much more effective than just lashing out.

Sharing with others, in a group situation, was particularly appreciated by some participants:

Emily: Substance misuse group is brilliant and everyone was so honest last week about where they were at, I found it very humbling and overwhelming the honesty in that group.

For others, one-to-one work was cited as the kind of support that had proven particularly effective:

Rose: I've been having counselling for quite a while and it's really beginning to help, because we're getting at the root of what the problem actually is. I've been allowed to go at my own pace which I feel is really good.

Family members and carers did not identify specific skills in the person they cared for, since coming to The Haven, but did cite an upsurge in motivation and a change in behaviour:

Rob: Since getting the help, she has got much, much better, and coming, she doesn't just come if she's in crisis, she comes and has a bed which she arranges in advance and uses that, and she really does work hard while she's here, talking and making use of everything that's here. She's doing things at home she wouldn't do before.

Sammy: I think it's been absolutely useful her being here, my wife. It's actually given her motivation that for many years prior to coming here, that we tried to get her to get up and do things. To actually see her wanting to do different things and actually doing different things indoors now is far better. It's the motivation we've been trying to give her for years.

Alex: The person hasn't changed, the behaviour has changed.

Tony: The self-harm and suicide attempts aren't as frequent.

Finally, one of the components participants spoke of in this theme was a growing self-awareness regarding both the source of their problems and their negative behaviours or ways of coping:

Charles: I've learned a lot about myself, that I've got problems in certain areas, sort of anger and stuff like that, and you know, alcoholism.

Katy: I've changed in lots of different ways and I've learned that the voices I hear are actually in my head.

Chloe: I actually feel that my behaviour has changed. It's become, in nursing jargon, more appropriate, it's less extreme, the majority of the time. I've self-harmed once, I've overdosed once, since you've been open and before it was numerous times. I'm now able to ask for help before I get to that stage. So I think that would say, perhaps, I am maturing a bit. My coping strategies are completely different now. I probably cope better than the average person on the street because I am more aware of triggers, I am more aware of negative coping, if you like, strategies rather than skills. I channel my feelings and emotions more constructively.

Hopes, dreams and goals

A sense of *hope* and realistic, attainable *dreams and goals* emerged as the next finding. Hope is a mysterious thing in that it can transcend life's catastrophes. Here some participants said they had begun to conceive of dreams and goals for the first time. Others began to link hope to a concept of the future and a range of specific dreams and goals began to be envisaged by participants.

The research group had highlighted this in their sub-analyses of categories and had discussed the unified theme at the research group meeting in March 2009. Finding hope is inherent within a number of levels of the pyramid, or hierarchy of progress, however, realistic dreams and goals began to find their place in the themes only after progress on the lower levels of the journey.

Early expressions of hope included statements about wanting to stay alive:

Stony: When I first attended The Haven I didn't like myself, I was wanting to commit suicide. I never thought anybody would like me or love me in any way. Now I don't even, I don't want to die.

May: Before The Haven I wanted to die. Now I want to live.

Some family members and carers also discussed issues of mortality:

Rob: It's keeping her alive. I don't think she would be alive without The Haven. I know with my wife, she didn't want to be around, so there was no tomorrow and now she has hope.

Sammy: We've had the conversation more than once, 'Yes I am glad I am now alive, I want to be alive now. I want to be well. I want to carry on living.'

Participants began to express the concept of hopes, dreams and goals in a very tentative way, often referring to the ability to simply get through the day:

Stony: I want to get on a bus and breathe at night without panic.

Sally: To be happy, lead a normal life, and come off all meds. I can only cope with one day at a time.

Christine: The dream for me is taking one day at a time.

Lucy: Trying to feel next week like I've felt this week.

Some participants highlighted the fact that hopes, dreams and goals were a new and, until now, alien concept:

Emily: Do you know what, I never dreamed I could have hopes and dreams and goals for the future until sitting with this lot.

Tiffany: I can only say that since I've come to The Haven that I've actually got hopes, goals and dreams, because I've never had them before.

Participants then began to link hope to a concept of the future:

Rose: I look to the future more than I ever did. It exists now. My vision has changed. I didn't even think about the future before I came here. It was as much as I could do to survive today. I hated the thought of tomorrow. I never wanted it to come.

Jonny: I think, well I know, I've survived it. The other thing is I think The Haven gives hope to everybody, that there's something better in the future. So you're not written off.

Leska: I actually thought that I have got a future now, it was really bleak before, but it actually looks like there is something now. Now, when I am just unconsciously sitting there, I do find myself wondering and thinking about the future.

Family members and carers also identified hope both within themselves and for those they care for:

Rob: I think hope. They have hope. She can see the future.

Sarah: They can see light at the end of the tunnel, they can see a bit of future really.

Sammy: Yes, I do have hope for the future.

However, one family member felt that hope had been lost and could not be invested in the future:

Tony: No, I'm so sorry, until (family member) puts drugs out of her life, no, none whatsoever. I'd love to be positive and, to be honest with you, it's hurt so much over the years I can't invest any more hope in (family member).

Initially, some client participants also felt devoid of hope:

Igor: I've got no dreams apart from nightmares.

Crystal: I've got no hopes dreams and goals. I feel empty inside.

Some espoused the desire to show others, who had harmed them, that they could progress in spite of this:

Boris: I have one goal I know I'll achieve and that's to turn around and say to all the fucking twats that have fucked up my life and say, fuck you, I've won, you've lost. If I can't achieve anything else in my life that's what I want to achieve and will achieve.

Leska: I'd like to be able to prove everybody wrong who said that I'd never get better and say, 'Fuck you,' really.

Over time, participants began to confidently and clearly define goals in education and for a career:

Ben: Since coming to The Haven I've had an idea implanted in my head to go back to university and I'm at the stage now where I'm getting the curriculum and believing I might be able to do it.

Alexis: I hope to do mathematics.

Poppy: My goal is to get through college and do my degree.

Katy: My goal is to go back and do my MA. That's my long-term goal.

Also, participants were very clear that, over time, their hopes, dreams and goals began to be more realistic:

Katy: My hopes and dreams are becoming a lot more realistic.

Elise: I think the biggest part of recovery certainly is actually learning to adapt to how the situation is in the real world. I've discovered there's a whole world of possibilities and employment prospects out there and it doesn't have to all centre around this sort of several walls The Haven is. I'd actually like to go and get a decent job and earn a reasonable amount of money so I can have a nice lifestyle to go with it.

Achievements

What participants felt they had accomplished emerged as a finding about *achievements*. This included both internal and external achievements. This interplay between the development of personal qualities, such as confidence and self-esteem, and their external expression, characterized their responses.

The importance of building practical skills which have a bearing on life outside The Haven was highlighted:

Sheila: I am learning to talk a bit more and that helps me outside. Just mundane things like going to the bank, I can actually speak to people behind the counter without just standing there and grunting at them.

Leska: One of the biggest new skills I'm learning is how to be a Mum, and I suppose another big skill I'm learning is to try and stand on my own two feet and try to deal with stuff, instead of asking The Haven for so much support, how to be patient, how to interact with someone who can't talk, and to love someone who's so dependent on you, learning to love you could say.

Jasmine: I never used to like going on public transport or getting in a car because of panic attacks, but since I've been here I've been able to get on trains and on the bus.

A sense of empowerment and having choices, and a voice, in relation to gaining confidence and self-esteem, were also cited as an achievement. The analogy of finding one's backbone was mentioned more than once:

Boris: I suppose the dominant skill I'm learning at The Haven is being more confident that I can achieve more than I think I can. I am stronger in my beliefs and I fight for what I think is correct.

103

Ross: It gives me support, boosts confidence and gives me something to focus on. The Haven, for me, it's like having an extra backbone.

Beginning from what was usually a high degree of self-loathing, during the course of the study, 75 per cent of client participants answering a question about their internal sense of self, reported positively regarding disliking themselves less. The majority who answered positively had been attending The Haven for two to three years:

Harry: I think I used to dislike myself a lot. I don't actually dislike myself now, although I dislike my behaviour at times, which is a massive difference and I'm actually able to go out and buy new clothes. So being able to spend money on myself has come from being at The Haven and being made to feel worthwhile.

Brunhilda: At The Haven you get so much positive feedback and just logically, if quite a lot of people think that you are a decent human being, logically you must be. Eventually, yes, you get re-programmed, it definitely does filter through.

Fred: I think how far I have come. When I think of that, I think no, I have done really well, and I know now, it's not an excuse, things that happened to me while I was in care and on the street, it wasn't my fault.

Chloe: There are things about myself that I do like. There are qualities and parts of my character that I think of as valuable and specific to me. So I value myself, so yes I do spend less time disliking myself.

This was sometimes combined with a sense of finding oneself, or 'the real me':

Rose: The change is due to actually learning who I am. I've been something else before now.

Donald: People have helped me to reach inside myself and get back to the cheeky little monkey.

The remaining 15 per cent of participants, who answered 'no' to the question about disliking oneself less, included some who had not been long in attendance at the service. Resistance to recovery is considered further in the next chapter in relation to four participants who had been at

The Haven for two to three years and, although other improvements had occurred, this did not yet include achieving a change in their internal sense of self:

Jasmine: No I still hate myself but my feelings here have changed, I'm not 136'd so often now, the police station used to be my second home.

Others spoke of achieving the confidence to start voluntary work, tackling stigma by training professionals, and reflected on not just having hopes, dreams and goals, but achieving them:

Poppy: I've done some volunteer work, and I've learnt that I am really good with animals.

Harry: My confidence has risen enormously. A year and a half ago I was never leaving the house. My hopes and dreams, they're not dreams anymore because I'm doing it with the Personality Disorder Awareness Program.

Still more spoke about their achievements in the different domains of social inclusion including activities aimed at tackling stigma and discrimination, finding a real home for the first time, discovering leisure activities, education and employment:

Boris: If by doing this exhibition we can change one person's opinions about personality disorder then we will have done some good.

Brunhilda: This is the first time I've had a place that feels like home. It's therapeutic in itself to be at home with my cat and potter about in the garden. I've never had a garden before. It's such an excellent de-stressor.

Poppy: I've been on theatre trips, Kew Gardens, Zoos, and Garden Centres, Wild Life Centres and other towns and cities like Norwich. It's just nice to have found friends who have the same interests. I feel more part of the outside community. I have widened my horizons and it has definitely increased my confidence and enjoyment in life.

Natasha: I started access planning and at first it was quite nerve wracking, sweaty palms, I could hardly hold a pen for the first two weeks. During the first week when I got home I had a panic attack. It's improved now and I'm starting to relax more easily. I feel good about it. I kind of feel proud I suppose, that I've managed to get this far. I am now on the access course and I've got an exam next week which means I'll be finished the first year.

Pablo: I've been on a hairdressing course for the last few months. To start with it was really difficult and this was the fourth or fifth time I've tried and never got past the second session, second minute! I'd just go in there and say…'Ah, I need the loo'… and I was gone. This time I went with the pain and the panic in a way. It's like a drama in your head, a self-whipped-up drama. I toughed it out this time. It's different when you're not influenced by any intoxicants in your system. I feel confident now. I just cut four people's hair this morning.

Tiffany: When I work with animals, I feel different, I know that I will not get any hassle, any abuse, I get unconditional affection and love which I sometimes do not get from my family. I had no purpose in life but over the two years of being here at The Haven and getting support and working with animals it has helped me to overcome my agoraphobia, my panic attacks.

Milly: I want employers to recognize that, given a supportive working environment, mental health service users are employable, reliable and responsible people. I feel it is now up to mental health service users to be more open and honest about their diagnosis and have a say. It is up to us who we tell and what we say but by being open and honest I feel I have started my journey of recovery.

Transitional recovery

The research group had begun to discuss the concept of *transitional recovery* at its meeting in September 2006 (Appendix II). Therefore, it was a concept that had been developing at The Haven for several years. By 2009, the consensus within the research group, at its meeting in May, was that this theme should form the final, and all embracing, apex of the pyramid. What transitional recovery means will become apparent as the ingredients of our discoveries about recovery are described below.

Although steps in the journey of recovery are expressed throughout the pyramid of progress, this theme concerns how participants defined recovery and shows the fears, barriers and progress on the journey. Some family members and carers expressed strong and clear opinions about the concept of recovery:

Sammy: Recovery is an individual thing. It is not necessarily, as a lot of professionals will lead you to believe, about getting a job. At the end of the day, for some people, it might just be getting out of the house for the first time in five years. It's an individual thing; it isn't a model, although some people try to tell you it is. It's a concept and it's an individual concept. It's not about government targets of getting a million people off of incapacity benefit. It's about a journey that somebody takes, and The Haven is assisting people in making that journey. Recovery is a goal for the individual and little steps along the way.

Dinah: I don't think recovery will ever be a position where you are declared well and put all this behind us, it won't be like that. I think this is going to be one of those things that will go through my partner's life forever and that certain trigger points, crisis points, certain issues will set her off again and we'll take a step back and there'll be times when we take a few steps forward and life's comparatively easy. How I define recovery for my partner is that she has her own life, and she feels capable of doing things outside, meeting friends, having a bit of a social life, where I'm not standing behind her propping her up. I think that will be recovery.

Rob: Once you start understanding what the problem is then you can start to work towards a better way of carrying on, mustn't say cure must we. I just think it's the individual thing. One thing I did think is there's no definition, but while they are moving forward they're in a state of recovery. If they keep moving that's good.

However, over 70 per cent of client participants felt that the concept of recovery was very frightening. Fear of failure was expressed:

Boris: I think recovery is frightening because for so long in my life I had so many people telling me I was never going to come to anything, spend my whole life in hospital. I am petrified that I am going to fail and I am going to prove everyone right. I sit there and I work on my journey to change things with the whole doubt in my head going, what happens if I don't achieve this, what happens if it goes wrong, what happens if I still go backwards?

Chloe: Success can be frightening. What if I fail?

A fear of the unknown was also cited by participants as a barrier to recovery:

Elise: I think there's an awful lot of people at The Haven that have lived in a world of inner torment for so long, and have lived a psychiatric based life for so long that to move away from that, even though they don't particularly like the life they have at the moment, but to move away from that and take on something new, with a whole new perspective and everything, it's always going to be scary. It's like moving to another country or a new flat. The change is what's so scary because it's so unpredictable.

Alexis: Extremely frightening! We're used to living with what is most familiar to us, it's our routine and it's what goes on day to day, month in, month out.

Eustace: Maybe the process towards it is frightening. Where does it lead you to?

Fear of the unknown was also described as being linked to a sense of identity, not knowing who 'the real me' is, and whether this will be acceptable to self and others:

Sally: Sometimes you don't know, it takes time to find out who you are and to start to try to change who you are. That takes quite a while.

Abigail: I find recovery is knowing yourself and it's very frightening because you're suddenly finding something that you have never known before and accepting them for who and what they are. I think the frightening thing is that you haven't got that person that's at the end of the line.

Boris: I know I am only the person I am due to where I've come from. I'd like to think that once I had recovered that I was always the same person but there's always that fear inside me that I might not be that person.

Milly: It's frightening for me because I don't know whether, by recovering, I'm going to lose my relationship, because I don't know whether my partner can accept me if I change.

Some participants made powerful statements about fear of recovery in relation to being defined by the diagnosis and a world of mental illness being all they had ever known:

Kim: Fucking scary, cos I've never known recovery. I've been in and out the system since 16.

Sheila: Yes, because it's all I've ever known, is this personality disorder, all this mental illness, ever since I was very young.

Some participants clearly stated that they felt it was too late for recovery and this barrier is discussed further in the next chapter:

Gemma: I think when you've spent half your life, it's a real struggle. I've found that, since the age of 14 when I started self-harming, over the years I have picked myself up, and now I have gone down again without realizing it. In the end you can be so sick and tired of the struggle. If I was 16 now I would not have gone backwards and forwards into hospital all my life. It would have made my life completely different if I'd had the understanding and not just be called attention seeking.

Abigail: Yes it's frightening, I can't change and I don't want to change.

Phoenix: I know a good line from a song which goes, 'dying is easy it's living that scares me to death', and I think that maybe says it for me.

Despite progress on the lower levels of the pyramid, significant barriers to the concept of recovery, as employment, were also highlighted by some participants in relation to risking what progress they had made:

Tiffany: I'm frightened of getting well then not being able to work. Like coming off benefits, that's what frightens me most.

Cosmic: At 51 to say that I've recovered is putting a hell of a lot at risk. I'll have to be forced out of this safety net, not that I'm lazy but I've got a dread of going back to what it was like before. I would overwork, do all the hours under the sun, then come down with depression and alcoholism. I might self-harm, then two weeks later get back on my feet and be able to do agency work, work myself to death again.

Brunhilda: I think recovery is frightening because in my imagination it means losing security that I've now got, which I've wanted for so long. I am aware that for a lot of the time nowadays I feel like I am in a comfort zone, but that's such a novelty, something that I've never experienced before.

One of the participants in the study, who was now working, confirmed that the world of paid employment can be a large leap to take:

Elise: Under the current benefits system you are either at work or on benefits, there doesn't seem to be anything in between. There have been some welfare rights concessions, but this needs to go much further. I could not have gone part-time and back to work gradually. I live on my own and organizing partial benefits isn't an option, yet a staged introduction to work would encourage many more to try it. Instead it's a complete paradigm shift. Where's the middle step?

Embarking on a road of recovery, possibly against the odds, some participants began to express excitement and desire, despite the fears and barriers:

Ian: At the beginning I think it is because it means you have to take a lot more responsibility and sometimes it's scary that people aren't around so much, and you have to deal with things a lot more on your own, but afterwards it makes you proud.

Curtis: I used to think it was frightening, because it's such a big step, but now I find I'm looking for it, I'm wanting it.

Rose: Yes I think it's frightening, but I also think it's exciting now.

This desire for recovery was highlighted by other participants as a key ingredient on the journey:

Charles: Wanting to do it is the main issue. There's nothing wrong with slipping back, it's trying to learn from it.

A recurring sub-theme in recovery for participants concerned fear of losing The Haven. This was expressed by family members and carers as a fear of the service losing funding, or getting too big, or clients getting too well and being asked to leave:

Rob: I always worry about The Haven being there. That it'll grow. Your community has a size at the moment that obviously works.

Sammy: I have a bit of a concern the person I care for expressed to me. What happens if The Haven sort of considers that she has got to a point where they can't help her anymore? The problem is what she's worried about is if she's been under mental health services for 30 years. I think this is the fear of, 'Well everyone perceives that I'm, you know, I don't need this anymore.'

Dinah: I do fear for the funding. You continue to get your funding and I know it's difficult in this economic climate. I've seen the economics cut £10,000 where it would save you £50,000 later.

Sarah: I would just say let's hope it carries on being here.

Client participants also expressed concern about losing The Haven and made it clear that progress could be greatly enhanced by knowing help is still on hand when needed:

Pablo: One of my first questions when I very first came here, I said, is this a conveyor belt to chuck us in and chuck us out, get us well, I said, or is this a firm base that stays here forever? Just hold my hand on my bad days. I hope that's not too much to ask.

One participant bravely voiced what we felt many Haven clients feared, that is, losing their base and the sense of home some had achieved for the first time in their lives:

Brunhilda: When I think of recovery I get very frightened because I think recovery is like being on the top of a mountain and if I've recovered it means that I won't need The Haven anymore, and I cannot imagine having no more contact with The Haven.

Because the word recovery could potentially become synonymous with the idea of loss, it became crucial to define the top of the mountain, or the apex of the pyramid, in a human and tenable way, that is, in a way that was going to work. As a result, the concept of *transitional recovery* was born, meaning that progress would be defined as a journey of small steps and progression would not be penalized by discharge, but rather rewarded by continued support. Remaining registered at the project, despite progress in the outside world, would also be contingent upon using the service less but knowing it still existed as a firm base:

Brunhilda: If you feel well-rooted then, like a tree, you can kind of branch out and blossom.

The Haven already espoused a philosophy of not rewarding negative behaviour, as described in the 'Learning the Boundaries' section of this chapter, and some participants also pointed out the necessity of focusing support on positive progress rather than creating dependency:

Cosmic: I think there's too many people that are not using self-management skills and becoming independent. I don't see The Haven as a place to land, it's a place to touch down and spring from.

Participants now began to define recovery as not necessarily being a cure or a loss of symptoms, but rather a realistic progression of small steps and achievable goals. They also began to describe their progress as a journey of recovery:

Elise: I think everybody's in recovery from the minute they enter the door way of The Haven, unless they desperately don't want to help themselves, because recovery is a journey and it starts with admitting that you've got the problem to be there in the first place.

Jenny: It's probably the hardest thing I think I have done in my life, and I'm not even there yet. I don't even know if I'm half way there. I don't even know what 'there' is like. I believe it's a journey, but I don't know if the journey ever ends.

Research participants now spoke of their progress in the clear knowledge that the concept of transitional recovery meant support would be ongoing, as they moved forward:

Doris: I love transitional recovery, I absolutely love it. I think it's the group I get the absolute most out of, and I know that quite a lot of people here feel the same. It's a very empowering group, it's a group that gives you a chance to move on; it helps give you the tools to move on. Since the social inclusion department has opened at The Haven I have been in college for almost a year and I have had considerable help from the transitional recovery tutor with my numeracy and I have passed my level two in this subject. Transitional recovery has aided in re-affirming my strengths in all areas of life.

Cosmic: I've learnt to take more risks lately, because I've got a safety net here, if things go wrong, there's people I can depend on.

Transitional recovery, as the apex of the pyramid, became a developmental and flexible concept, where clients could continue their journey of recovery by defining and pursuing their unique goals and dreams, and where they had a choice about whether to remain registered at The Haven. Transitional recovery, as the apex of Figure 5.1 (on page 81), embraces the whole pyramid of progress.

CHAPTER 6

Analysis of the Journey of Recovery

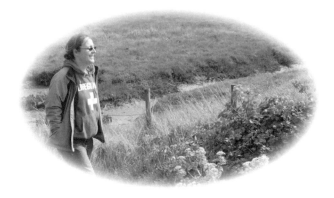

I spent years of my life wanting to be in hospital because I thought it would bring me more sympathy and more love and attention. I know that I get more love and attention now because I've got well and I've actually developed a life and people are interested in that life. It's an ongoing process; you never actually get there. You are always recovering. For me recovery has been able to actually function on my own, with minimal support, because of the things I've learnt. I'm well into recovery because I've actually developed enough internalized strategy in my brain to cope with things.

Service User Quotation

Our conceptual map of the journey of recovery is the pyramid illustrated in the last chapter (Figure 5.1, page 81). Now each level of the pyramid is analyzed in sequence, from the base upwards, and this represents a synthesis of the recovery concept, as a way of understanding the process of recovery for people with a personality disorder diagnosis.

Attachment and trust

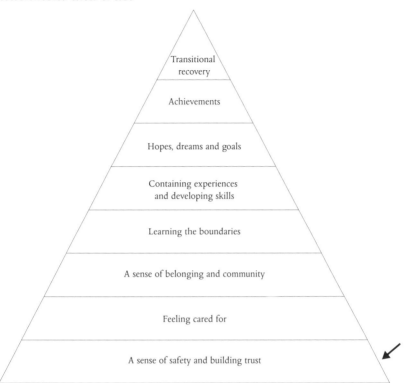

Figure 6.1 The pyramid of recovery:
A sense of safety and building trust.

Basic trust is associated with secure attachment. Campling (1999) proposes that severe personality disorder is related to insecure and disorganized attachment, where an infant may freeze on separation and be unable to sustain organized patterns of behaviour. She suggests that such experiences yield a future generation of people with personality disorder. Therefore, in working with someone who has a personality disorder diagnosis, trust has to be created in a very tangible way. In this study *a sense of safety and building trust* emerged as the foundation stone on which progress could be built.

When individuals began to feel safe at The Haven and to start to build trust they had entered a safe environment, a sanctuary, and they became part of a containing group (Bloom 1997). The Haven aspired to be such a sanctuary, a place of refuge and protection. Participants expressed the tangibility of the sense of safety they experienced:

Gemma: When I've felt really vulnerable or in a crisis all the staff, I can't say anyone who hasn't, have made me feel secure, safe and put me at ease and just give me that secure feeling and I can't find the words, strength and courage, sort of, to face things you know, and the effort has still been there whilst I'm trying to do it, carrying that out.

Leska: When I've been feeling vulnerable I've always had someone come to talk to me, been reassured that I am safe, and that there are people here to support me and I'm not alone.

Predictability and consistency appeared to be important ingredients, as was availability evidenced by participants highlighting the fact that The Haven would be there 24 hours a day. The 24/7 availability of the service was explicitly given the highest rating by participants, at 28 per cent in answer to the question about how The Haven helps them, and it was implicit in other responses. It existed as an object even when someone was not present at the service:

Poppy: If you are in crisis, knowing that you can phone up and get help. Knowing that there is people here, then you can feel safe.

Intensity of emotional pain and fragility of identity require a leap of faith on the part of an individual to reach out for help. Knowing that somewhere is safe and that people there can be trusted is a necessary enabler:

Fred: I used not to talk, it made me vulnerable in speaking, you know, you are opening yourself up for ammunition or further abuse, but I'm learning to trust more, and to ask for help.

The basis of a safe world is founded on the ability of care-givers to be there for a baby or child throughout episodes of unbounded distress and intolerable feelings (Haigh 1999). Winnicott (1971) describes a secure child as one who is able to express destructive emotions, 'Hello object, I will destroy you.' Consistency and containment are cited as essential to the therapeutic alliance. In a therapeutic community this is a fundamental component of the therapeutic milieu. Here, safety and trust are generated when primitive feelings are re-experienced and are accepted without rejection. This is the foundation for a safe world where one can survive:

Boris: It's through this place I've learnt that I don't have to hide my problems. I don't have to hide behind a smile anymore. I can come in and I can cry and I can be me for once, something I haven't done for years, you know, and I can do it being safe.

> I'm given time, that's all I need and that gives me the ability to trust again.

Aiyegbusi and Norton (2009) describe the function of containment in a hospital inpatient ward as maintaining physical well-being, relieving someone of the burden of self-control and temporary removal from the stressors of the outside world. However, they highlight the likelihood of suppressing the patient's own initiative and magnifying feelings of hopelessness. Conversely, an authentic sense of safety and trust is described by participants in this study as generating an increased ability to take risks and a new ability to talk instead of engaging in self-destructive behaviour:

Rose: It makes me feel safer which helps me take more risks than I ever have. It's really working, I've learned to trust which enables me to talk instead of taking things out on myself.

Creating a culture of warmth

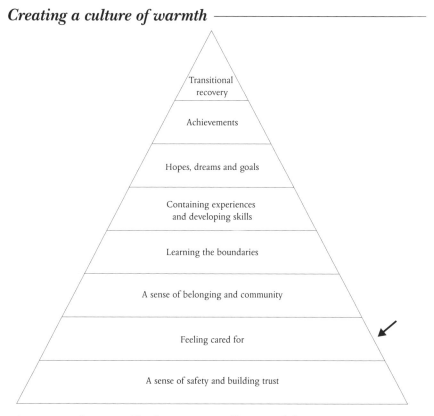

117

Figure 6.2 The pyramid of recovery: Feeling cared for.

The word *care* is common parlance in the psychiatric arena; 'community care'; 'the care program approach'; 'care planning'; 'aftercare'; 'evidence-based care'; 'secure care'; 'quality of care'. But what does *care* mean? The Oxford Dictionary definition of care is: 'Serious attention and thought; to be concerned or interested'. The concept of *feeling cared for*, the second step in our pyramid of progress, also suggests warmth, comfort, nurture and being valued.

It has been suggested that care is not necessarily consistent with a therapeutic community approach and that self-reliance should be the emphasis, rather than making cups of tea for clients or always responding to their pain with soothing words (Tucker 1999). It is true that at The Haven, facing the enormity and complexity of problems, care was not always a sentimental concept. In addition to warmth, other responses were also called for, such as toughness, consistency and honesty. However, The Haven may have differed from some therapeutic communities in that participants in the study clearly defined what they felt were the component parts of feeling cared for and expressed their need for, and deep appreciation of such responses and the relationship this had to the first step of the pyramid, building trust.

The staff team at The Haven, from the administrator and housekeeper to volunteers and the clinical staff, all understood the vital importance of first contact. The warm welcome and friendliness at The Haven was a frequent cause for comment by visitors, including family members and carers:

Sarah: I have to say that I just think The Haven is just a calm, happy, just a caring place.

Participants emphasized first contact responses:

Jonny: Last week I wasn't well and I get somebody from The Haven on the door. It's just, they care, and that matters one hell of a lot.

Participants rated the caring nature of The Haven second highest, at 22 per cent, in their answers to the question about how The Haven helps them, and this was implicit in many other responses:

Sally: When I have been really down I have been taken into a room and they have made me a cup of coffee and they wouldn't let me out of the door until I have got myself together.

Creating a culture of care in terms of warmth and kindness becomes how a place is. Thoughtfulness and kindness can be infectious and, if clients are treated well, they in turn treat others well and the atmosphere becomes one of warmth and care:

Doris: I think a lot of people here realize what it's like to be lonely. We all know what it's like so we all make an extra effort to be friendly, to be nice; to make a cup of tea.

Being believed in and encouraged are crucial ingredients for recovery (Turner-Crowson and Wallcraft 2002). Aiyegbusi and Norton (2009) suggest that validation may take many forms, including the kind of attention that can affirm someone's importance and individuality. Clients in the study cited instances of being listened to and valued as important aspects of feeling cared for:

Doris: They make you feel that, for half an hour, you are the sole focus of their attention. You're not just a number and you've got these issues and they are going to sit there and listen to you. Even if it goes over, they are not clock-watching. There's no 'I'm going to get my lunch now.' You are important.

119

What it means to belong ————————————————————

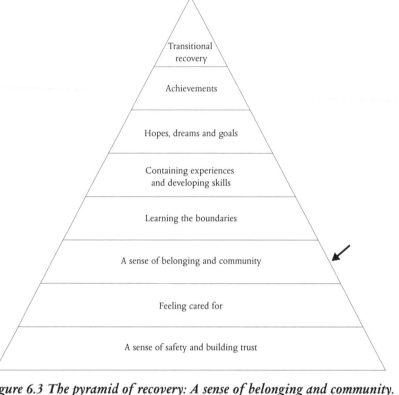

Figure 6.3 The pyramid of recovery: A sense of belonging and community.

The first of the five key principles of a therapeutic community is described by Rapoport (1960) as 'attachment and a culture of belonging'. Secure early attachment gives an infant a consistent experience of existence, which is internalized and provides a greater ability to face later life experiences (Bowlby 1969). When emotional development has not provided secure attachment for a child, the first step in treatment is to recreate that secure attachment (Haigh 1999). The first two steps on our pyramid of recovery had already begun to construct attachment in terms of safety and trust, and feeling cared for. The third step, *a sense of belonging and community*, is where clients, who had experienced a history of abuse or trauma and poor relationships, began to value being part of something. This third level of the pyramid is related to the two levels below, in that trust and feeling cared for are experienced as a reciprocal relationship that reinforces a sense of being part of something and belonging.

Shared experiences and common ground were aspects of community highlighted by participants as something which made them feel understood. This gave them a sense of being somewhere they felt they belonged, often for the first time:

Cosmic: I feel more secure. I used to feel like a freak. Why am I so different from the neighbours? But this is a whole club full of them and I keep in mind that I'm not alone.

Wilf: You can see by some people that they have been as low as you have. We've all been down right to that bottom, you know, well, hell really isn't it, and then some of us more than once. It helps you talk to people because they've been through the same sort of pain.

Winnicott (1965) suggests that a facilitating environment acts as a container where the gap between the container and the contained starts to open up and the individual can begin to explore autonomous identity:

Doris: What I have found is that other people can like me. I am less serious. I have rediscovered my sense of humour and I have rediscovered my ability to make other people laugh. I rediscovered the fact I am good. I am not as bad as I think I am. If someone is feeling rubbish I will give them a cup of tea, give them a kind word, give them a hug.

Clearly voicing their newly developed experience of healthy attachment, participants defined The Haven community as giving them a sense of home and family:

Poppy: I'm now learning to use The Haven to help myself and it's like an extended family that I haven't got really.

Leska: The Haven community, it means a lot to me, it's like having a family all under one roof.

Love is not enough

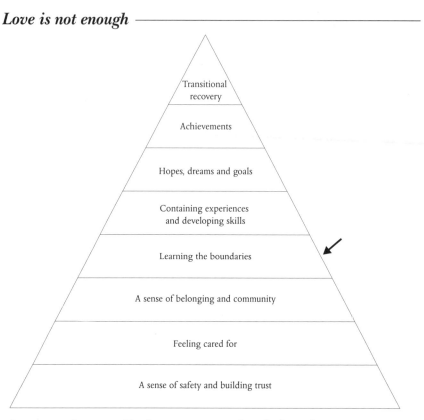

Figure 6.4 The pyramid of recovery: Learning the boundaries.

On the first three steps of the pyramid, in the stages of the journey of recovery at The Haven, healthy attachment was built within a culture of safety, warmth and belonging. Norton and Bloom (2004) emphasize the importance of ensuring that the culture of a therapeutic community is not eroded by difficult behaviours, suggesting that tolerance should have its limits. This brings us to the fourth level of the pyramid, *learning the boundaries*.

For someone who has experienced early attachment difficulties, healthy attachment may be longed-for but also feared. The concept of attachment becomes idealized as an individual yearns for unconditional love. Haigh (1999) describes this process as a journey through the developmental phases of attachment in a therapeutic community. As an individual struggles with sadness, fear, pain and anger, savage mechanisms can sometimes come into play. The ability to be honest may be blocked by feelings of shame and humiliation. Here, denial, lying, projection and splitting begin to be demonstrated. Someone may display unconscious impulses to envy, spoil, steal or destroy what is good:

Brunhilda: Community isn't all about harmony and everyone loving each other and that sort of thing, because life is full of challenges and difficulties and rubbish and so inevitably that comes up within the community.

Living too long with untenable emotions and in a state of chronic hyper-arousal, people with a personality disorder diagnosis also frequently adopt dysfunctional behaviours to numb unbearable feelings and to swiftly bring their mood down to a manageable level. Hurting the body can create temporary calm because of endorphin release. Such behaviours include self-harm and substance misuse. This is how people have coped and, for many, they become deeply ingrained coping strategies. Although containment is achieved through holding someone's distress, that distress may trigger unacceptable behaviours. Bettleheim (1950) suggests that love is not enough and that the damaging expression of pain needs containing measures. To create psychological safety at The Haven these self-destructive behaviours needed to be actively challenged. An approach to people's capacity to create negative effects for others must be effective. All this represents boundary setting and the social and moral limits that need to be present to create a safe community. Whatever rules and boundaries are negotiated in an organization, the vital issue is that the boundaries are clear to everyone and that they are agreed, known and understood:

123

Charles: To help support me in my recovery I'd rather have clear guidelines and boundaries, so I know where I am coming from. The rules are here for a reason, and they weren't just put here for the sake of putting here, they were put here to keep everybody safe and they do serve that role.

The process of democratically setting and applying boundaries is cited by Hinshelwood (1996) as a learning process which addresses respect, not just for the reality of self, but also for the reality of others, enabling an individual to ultimately find the self as the seat of agency and to begin to take control and responsibility. Once more, the interrelationship between layers of the pyramid is highlighted as clients begin to take responsibility, not just for their own behaviour, but also for the behaviour of others:

Boris: Community is about treating other people as you would like to be treated yourself. The urge to do destructive things to yourself takes over. When very strong boundaries are imposed it's the respect that we have for The Haven that stops us from breaking them. This makes you go to staff to ask for help rather than going down that destructive path.

In terms of primitive emotions and behaviours, Campling (1999) proposes that it may be more difficult to destroy a group. She also suggests that clients are often in a better position to inject realism into such situations:

Doris: We understand why people want to come in, for example, under the influence. We understand the struggle and the difficulties but we have, on those occasions, stood together as a community and we have said, 'This is unacceptable.' People aren't abandoned at such difficult times, but the learning is about what is acceptable and unacceptable to the community and what is healthy and positive for the individual. We all take responsibility for The Haven community but, at the end of the day, the message is that each person has to take responsibility for themselves, with our support.

Evidencing the efficacy of learning the boundaries, and supporting service users in deciding what those boundaries should be, over two-thirds of participants in the study reported a reduction in their use of negative coping strategies:

Elise: I have had the whole urges to cut when I've felt low. I think, like an alcoholic, once things go wrong you resort to things you knew once worked. I have sort of redressed this. A lot of the reason has been because of the ruling about coming in when you have cut, or coming in when you have drunk alcohol. So you have to respect the values of the place. I now don't cut. To me to cut would be such a backward step I don't even want to go there.

Recreating healthy attachment and opening the door to therapeutic work

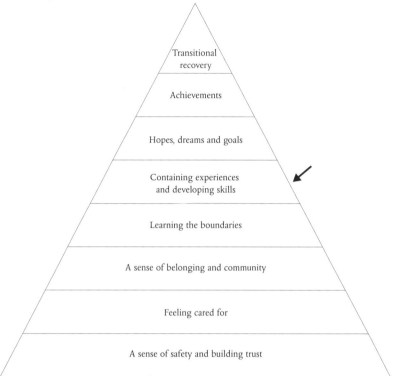

Figure 6.5 The pyramid of recovery:
Containing experiences and developing skills.

The first four steps in the hierarchy of progress have aimed to develop healthy attachment in terms of safety, and trust, feeling cared for, a sense of belonging and learning acceptable boundaries, limits and behaviour. This is how participants at The Haven described their journey through the developmental phases of recreating attachment. It was not until a degree of stable progress had been made, in terms of healthy attachment that clients began to advance to the level where they were *containing experiences and developing skills*. This constituted the creation of what might be called 'readiness'. In the preceding chapter, Figure 5.2 (page 96) graphically represents the journey on the upper levels of the pyramid as being supported by the foundation pillars of the first four levels. This provides answers to why someone with a personality disorder diagnosis may be progressing, or why someone may not.

In a client group desperately in need of therapy, trust can be so low, and behaviour so chaotic, risky and destructive, that meaningful therapy cannot take place. Having a history and pattern of expressing distress destructively in mainstream services, this type of presenting scenario existed for some new clients for a period of time after joining The Haven. Feelings of unworthiness meant that some found they were unable to ask for help, resulting in crisis presentations such as overdoses and self-harm. As progress was achieved on the first four levels of the pyramid, the overwhelming desire to become free from unbearable feelings, by acting them out, was replaced by the ability to reach out for help, talk and re-channel feelings, as described by one participant below:

Fred: I'm also clean and have stayed clean. Kind of like instead of popping a pill, I come here. Stopping drugs, feeling the emotion and learning from it.

The Haven's recovery ethos had an underpinning therapeutic approach, as a psychoanalytic therapeutic community arising from attachment theory. Staff and clients also employed an additional variety of approaches with therapies in group and individual work. As clients progressed on the lower levels of the pyramid, various groups and one-to-one support existed at the service:

Natasha: It's just that there's something to do all the time. They encourage you to do things but there's no pressure.

Cosmic: The groups are excellent, the way you can just turn up for a group, I find that very supportive. I know that's in my diary, I like the group, and I turn up.

Charles: I've been using the one-to-ones. It's a way forward for me if I'm feeling angry I vent my anger.

A dialectical behaviour therapy (DBT) skills group existed where group members could work together to achieve a life worth living. Although there was no dedicated DBT therapist for individual work at The Haven, one-to-one support, or reinforcement, came from the team as a whole, where contact was available on a 24-hour, seven days a week basis:

Natasha: I find DBT's been very helpful especially with negative thoughts and coping skills, mindfulness.

Additionally, the life skills program taught at The Haven covered skills such as anxiety management, anger management, assertiveness and confidence building, and tools to reduce self-harm, eating distress and substance misuse. Life skills incorporated features from the WRAP program, 'wellness recovery action plan' (Copeland 2001) where individuals could explore their own repertoire of wellness, or recovery tools such as sleep, good nutrition, self-soothing activities and uplifting pursuits. The life skills program was developed to involve less commitment than the DBT skills group, because it was a rolling program where clients could attend missed sessions and re-do the program, or selected sessions from it:

Cosmic: The life skills is brilliant because it's so varied, and I've learned a lot and it's good to be re-running the course as well, because if there's anything that I've missed, or wasn't paying attention.

As skills were built at groups such as DBT and life skills, a range of individual therapies also took place, provided by Haven staff and sessional counsellors. Approaches ranged from psychodynamic to cognitive, with the emphasis on the therapeutic relationship. The experience of therapy also highlights the interrelationship between levels of the pyramid when therapeutic work may have a profound effect on feelings, and apparent setbacks may occur:

127

Harry: I've been learning where a lot of my difficulties have stemmed from which is, hopefully, in the long term, helping me to overcome them. At the moment my self-harm has got a lot worse. But I'm going through a very difficult period at the moment and the thing I have to realize is that, although I'm getting less judgemental of other people, I'm getting more judgemental with myself. So I'm actually, at the moment, more likely to self-harm but I'm less likely to get myself into a fight with someone else.

Young *et al.* (2003) appeared to have very clearly identified the maladaptive schemas we were working with on a daily basis at The Haven. Although a small number of staff members received some schema therapy training, the clinical team, as a whole, identified threads of the schema approach throughout much of their work with clients. Motivational Interviewing

(Rollnick, Miller and Butler 1995) was used by some staff, along with neurolinguistic programming, NLP (O'Connar 2001), and trauma incident reduction, TIR (French and Harris 1998). TIR combines engagement with acceptance and commitment to psychological flexibility. This is another approach which blends aspects of CBT, DBT, schema therapy and mindfulness (Kabat-Zinn 2001). Staff and clients worked together with a variety of overlapping approaches that reinforced progress on the first four levels of the pyramid, *developing skills* and helping clients to begin to *contain experiences*. From a position of trust meaningful therapy began to occur:

Rose: The counselling I'm receiving, I have been for quite a while, is just fantastic. I had ten years of psychotherapy and I still managed to avoid the issues. With the counselling I think it's the fact that it's here. It makes me feel safer which makes me take more risks than I ever have.

Participants also began to express a new ability to mentalize; to separate out from their mental processes and reflect on them (Bateman and Fonagy 2004). Experiences began to be remembered, understood and contained and skills developed to start to enable that person to function more rationally and effectively:

Elise: I've got the ability to think things through, to actually find my own solutions. I've developed a more logical mind.

Hope and its relationship to recovery

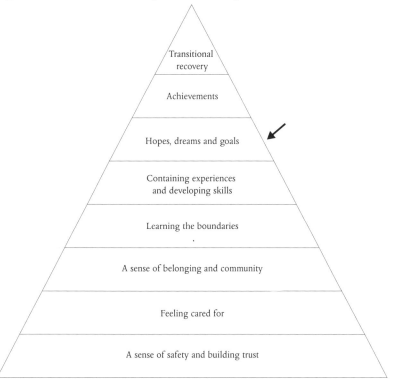

Figure 6.6 The pyramid of recovery: Hopes, dreams and goals.

Mental health, like many conditions in the health arena, is subject to a cure-based approach. Although dealing with symptoms and developing skills had an important place in the journey, they were not an underpinning principle in the user-defined concept of recovery. Waiting until all symptoms have subsided, before trying to discover and use one's abilities, could take a very long time and hope for a cure can overtake other ambitions (Repper and Perkins 2003):

Ross: We spend too much time looking for a cure when there is none, we can only learn to live alongside our illnesses by re-thinking the way we think to re-train the way we go about our daily lives and to learn to use our past experiences to guide us to where we want to be in life rather than carrying on the way we do.

Davidson (2003) talks of living outside mental illness and the importance of not being defined by illness but rather renewing *hope* and believing in a renewed sense of self:

Brunhilda: Is personality disorder an illness or a disability? Because, if it's an illness, there's a possibility of a cure but, if it's a disability then the way to approach it, just as it is of a physical disability, is that it's possible to learn to live a fruitful life.

Coleman's (1999) message of hope is about creating a capacity for recovery out of mental illness and distress. The importance of hope, and the idea that someday things will get better, is cited by Deegan (1988) as the essential ingredient for those who are recovering. Anthony (1993) proposes that recovery is possible even when symptoms and disabilities continue. Here, illness and wellness are seen as independent variables where new meaning and purpose are sought in the face of the effects of mental illness (Roberts and Wolfson 2004).

A focus on a deficit in skills can create a sense of hopelessness which is a feeling easily triggered in the face of past trauma. Deegan (1990) characterizes this 'giving-up', indifference and apathy as a way of surviving and protecting the last vestiges of the wounded self:

Fred: Things that have happened to me when I was in care and on the street, the world I was in before was so black, and that was hard, I was petrified of becoming well and then failing every time, failing myself again, I just couldn't take that anymore.

When someone has been repeatedly traumatized, or subjected to an environment that is sufficiently out of their control, they will give up trying to make changes (Bloom 1997). Experiences within the mental health system may have compounded such learned helplessness:

Abigail: I can't change and I don't want to change.

Even when support and skills training are offered someone may feel unable to make use of them:

Ben: I find the life skills group very threatening, so much so I haven't been able to sit through a whole one yet. I've hung on to my coping strategies which are distinctly negative because I feel that if I give them up them I'm lost. All my one-to-ones are spent with me blubbing and them offering me tissues.

The fostering of autonomy for each individual necessarily becomes vitally important. Repper and Perkins (2003) describe this as inspiring the hope, confidence and trust needed to activate the internal resources necessary to conceive of and pursue *dreams and goals*. However, being believed in and encouraged and the importance of support and friendship, interdependence and connectivity, in the early stages of recovery, are cited as crucial in helping to break the cycle of despair (Turner-Crowson and Wallcraft 2002; Russinova 1999). The earlier steps on the pyramid of progress have embodied this type of caring and encouraging approach at The Haven, which generated feelings of mutuality of trust, being cared for and belonging:

Sheila: It's a lot friendlier. It's a lot more caring and it's also trusting. It trusts me a lot more than other services, and you don't get talked down to and treated as though you are some kind of idiot.

Cosmic: I've had the confidence to start voluntary work because you had the confidence in me to show me the advert, see, for the job, so there.

Peer support and inspiration are also crucial ingredients in this activation of hopes, dreams and goals:

Wilf: Seeing the people who have moved on to college and stuff, you can set yourself a little goal then, can't you. They've done it, so you know, maybe there's a chance.

Milly: I think that the transitional recovery group gives you a lot of hope.

Coleman (1999) believes that recovery depends on self-help and collaboration. Perkins (1999) suggests that, in their support, services should shift their focus to the unique nature of the individual journey that each person travels. Nehls (2000) highlights the significant challenges for people who have attracted a personality disorder diagnosis in terms of stigma and the guarded prognosis of professionals. She calls for a fundamental shift, away from pessimism and paternalism, towards a new vision of services constructed by the consumer. The hope-inspiring environment at The Haven was intrinsically designed to share power and restore control to its users, both in terms of how the service was set up and run and how research was conducted:

131

Boris: The Haven is completely different to any other service I have ever used. In every other service you don't actually have an opinion or your voice isn't heard. At The Haven your voice is heard and your opinions taken into consideration, and everyone is treated individually here and you're not a number anymore here, you're your own person.

Brunhilda: I think it's great the way clients take such a part in research and setting parameters and policies.

In terms of hopes, dreams and goals, the importance of balancing realism with optimism is stressed (Repper and Perkins 2003). Research participants were clear that, over time, their aspirations began to be more realistic:

Chloe: Everyone has the potential in them to succeed, but it's about taking it each step at a time. It's about setting achievable goals.

Pursuing aspirations requires taking risks and Repper and Perkins (2003) also suggest that the ability to accept setbacks, and an uncertain future, is a significant challenge and an essential part of creating hope-inspiring relationships:

Doris: Recovery is like a road, a country road that's full of speed bumps and windy corners, and you travel along it and you think, yea you're getting somewhere, then you go over a bump and you get set back a bit, but you have to keep going and eventually you'll get to the end of the road and you'll find another road that goes somewhere that might be less bumpy.

Hope is also linked to taking control and responsibility over one's problems and life (Repper and Perkins 2003; Turner-Crowson and Wallcraft 2002). Deegan (1988) and Allott, Loganathan and Fulford (2003) describe an attitude, an approach to life, and a moment or turning point in relation to becoming unstuck and beginning to take that control:

Doris: All the help in the world is great but you have got to want to get to where you want to be. It's nothing you can be shown. You have just got to get your own fight back.

Identity and roles

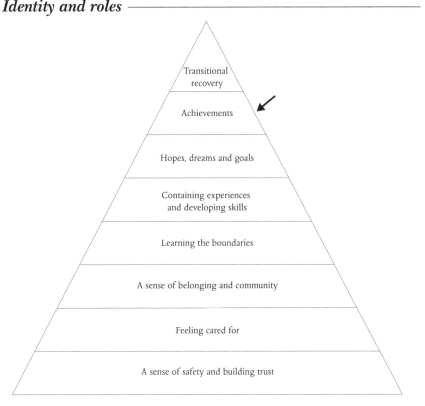

Figure 6.7 The pyramid of recovery: Achievements.

Identity and valued roles are central to *Achievements* and to giving meaning to life. Deegan (1993) talks of people's contributions that we can perceive and value, but she suggests that learning to value oneself is the real challenge. Supporting recovery is about helping people to build self-esteem and identity and to find valued roles in society (Allott *et al.* 2003). The findings in the previous chapter highlighted 'disliking oneself less' as a starting point in what was often a high degree of self-loathing. Thirty-six out of 48 participants responded positively to the question, 'Since coming to The Haven do you spend less time disliking yourself?' The majority had been attending The Haven for two to three years, suggesting that building self-esteem, even in a hope-inspiring environment, takes time:

Christine: I think the biggest lesson that this place has to teach you is self-acceptance because so many people here accept us then sometimes I look and think eh, how? Why? But then you transfer that on yourself and you then learn different ways of coping.

A sense of identity accompanied new found self-esteem and confidence:

Leska: I've started to find my identity and I've started to live life again.

However, four respondents who had been attending The Haven for two to three years answered no:

Sally: I still dislike myself. I don't know if it will ever change, it's always as far as I can remember for such a long time ago, that's just how I feel about myself.

Roberts and Wolfson (2004) talk of the dynamics of resistance in recovery. Aspects of lack of progress for some participants did not always show in research responses and one dimension that emerged is what Bartlett (1932) describes as the phenomenon of people making sense of something retrospectively. In psychological terms he called this 'effort after meaning'. This search for explanations for current conditions may involve rationalizations. We had participants who, after joining The Haven, had disclosed a history of sexual or other abuse for the first time. However, we also had those who appeared to fabricate early abuse or claim they had been subject to recent trauma such as being raped, when this was not in fact true. Such 'effort after meaning' presented explanations that might be commensurate with the pain and symptomatology being experienced by someone, but this did not open the door to meaningful progress. Staff considered it to be a mark of developing trust and progress when such rationalizations were eventually disclosed by the client as fabrications. They were never disclosed at research events, not even in the privacy of an individual interview. This is likely to be because of the shame associated with disclosing such fabrications and the need for the safety of an individual therapy session in which to do so. However, one carer did allude to such fabrications:

Tony: She invents things. Try to get to the root of it, because obviously my (family member) is in crisis for a reason, and rather than dealing with the reason she's making one up.

Another clinical facet of rationalization constitutes a very difficult and costly dimension of this client group and is characterized as MUS, medically unexplained symptoms (HMSO 2009). Physical illness for people with mental health problems occurs at significantly higher rates than in the general population. Lowered immune systems, due to extended periods of depression, accounted for some of this amongst our participants. Also, self-neglect, constituting more subtle forms of self-harm had exacerbated conditions such as asthma. Some participants had encountered genuine and significant health difficulties during the course of the study, such as cancer and chronic anaemia. Two older respondents died before the end of the study, both of natural causes related to cardiovascular problems. It was to be expected that general health would improve over time as respondents progressed on their journey of recovery. In Chapter 5, tables of service and cost-savings show some degree of reduction in the use of primary care and general hospital admissions. However, medically unexplained physical symptoms (MUS) existed to a significant degree. This included conditions such as pseudo fits, intermittent wheelchair and crutch use, which caused irritation to some who genuinely needed to use such aids, and other conditions that showed no medical basis when subject to tests. Although this issue was not brought up at research events, the research group originated the subject for discussion more than once as noted in research diary minutes for May and June 2009, Appendix II.

Being party to the conversations at the group meetings, I can relate that research group members felt there was a section of clients who were very stuck in a sick role. This did not concern only mental health difficulties, and having become defined by one's diagnosis, it also concerned physical illness, and some of this was considered to be spurious by research group members. MUS remained a significant challenge, particularly in terms of clarifying whether physical symptoms had a foundation or not. This was because those with mental health problems can often have genuine physical health problems, erroneously ascribed to mental illness, and have a much higher rate of mortality than the general population of the same age groups. The staff team continued to work therapeutically with the underlying issues for those with MUS, whilst being careful not to reward lack of progress with too much attention. In the meantime, to save time and costs, there was an effort to try to avoid unnecessary health-care referrals where possible, such as calling ambulances unnecessarily. Adshed and Jacob (2009) suggest that people with personality disorders have difficulties in effectively obtaining care from others. Related to early experiences with their carers, this can result in a tendency to try to elicit care in coercive ways.

The concept of resistance can move beyond learned helplessness, and the time and patience required in beginning to support people to feel cared for, valued and empowered to make choices. The process of recovery is sometimes fraught with complex losses. Gregory (2004) outlines what he considers to be the four thematic stages in the treatment of borderline personality disorder. Stage one mirrors the early steps in our pyramid in that issues of feeling safe are cited. Gregory then discusses a second stage, a dichotomy, where someone may exist in a state of inner conflict about whether they are a victim or a guilty perpetrator. This internal split is a response to severe trauma. The person may think about how they were abused, neglected or abandoned and consider themselves a victim. Or they may believe themselves to be evil because this would not have happened unless they were bad. Who is to blame? There is nothing fair about trauma, which is tragic and does not imply someone must have done wrong in order to experience it. Third, traumatized children may also sacrifice their sense of worth in an attempt to maintain a vision of their care-givers as good. This internal conflict can be very difficult to resolve because the person is unable to make sense of their experience, and Gregory considers this to be the most prolonged stage of recovery. He proposes that the next stage of the process of recovery concerns issues about grieving the loss of long and closely held views and fantasies, and worries about self-worth. Giving up a fantasy that care-givers or perpetrators were good is a loss and grieving process. Fears of separation, of becoming detached and alone, can also be present. The client may experience an undermining of progress from family members during this stage as old patterns of relating are challenged. Roberts and Wolfson (2004) also consider that symptoms carry significant meanings for people and that part of the process of resolution may involve deep loss and grieving. This is related to sense of identity where a world of illness and psychiatric labelling may be all that person has ever known, resulting in spoiled identity (Goffman 1963):

Ben: Personality disorder is all I've got and if you take that away there'll be nothing left.

Another approach to mental illness or disorder might involve what Tait, Birchwood and Trower (2003) call 'sealing over'. They suggest that, for those experiencing psychosis, there can be a recovery-style where a sufferer may decide that, despite illness, they want to forget about it and move on.

The Tait study showed that insight is not necessarily linked to 'sealing over' as a recovery-style and, therefore, is not synonymous with denial. They advocate interventions tailored to a recovery-style which minimizes the risk of deterioration in the absence of long-term treatment. Not overtly defining 'treatment', their paper also does not exclude medication as its definition. However, Harding *et al.* (1987), in their seminal study, claim recovery levels of two-thirds of people suffering from schizophrenia followed up over more than 30 years. Although not about personality disorder, this study is cited here because it evidences significant claims, for 68 per cent, about freedom from medication as a given. This proposes a revolutionary concept that people with schizophrenia may eventually recover and may become medication free. The National Institute for Health and Clinical Excellence advises that, in the treatment of borderline personality disorder, medication should be for short-term crisis use only, favouring psychological treatments (NICE 2009).

So, where does this leave the person who has attracted a diagnosis of personality disorder? Are their achievements built on psychological progress or do they stem from hope and self-belief, or both? The disenchanted words of one research participant follow:

Stony: The Haven as a community isn't that good really, to be honest, because people are, like I said over again, focusing on the actual illness rather than trying to move forward with everything, and everybody's competing on how ill they are rather than trying to be better.

Stony decided not to dwell on the past and resented those who seemed to be doing so. With permission from Stony, I have included some details of this person's story and the progress made.

After a number of years in secure hospitals, due to life-threatening self-harm, Stony started to attend Haven groups and was then discharged from hospital. Independent living followed and a reuniting with siblings, then a fiancée emerged, however, Stony still struggled with agoraphobia but maintained a cheerful outlook on life. Then came a break-up with the fiancée and Stony experienced a re-emergence of untenable feelings and difficult behaviour. After swallowing a razor blade Stony fortunately came straight to The Haven, was assessed there by the mental health team, and had a subsequent two-week stay in the psychiatric acute inpatient ward. This was the first hospitalization for almost four years.

During the hospital admission Stony had leave and came to a Haven life skills session and said, for the first time, that psychological therapy was the way forward. Once discharged from hospital, therapy began at The Haven. However, feelings unearthed during the therapy proved too painful and Stony decided not to attend for more sessions at that time. Bearing in mind that this person's history includes, during time in care, being chained with a sibling while being systematically sexually abused, it is not difficult to appreciate how untenable those emotions proved to be. But what courage Stony showed in pursuing life with hope and achieving some dreams. Physical appearance and presentation became pleasant and well-groomed, an unrecognizable comparison to the Stony who was in a secure hospital. Stony continues to hope and to achieve aspirations and dreams and whether this will include psychological therapy is a very personal choice. Bettleheim (1960) claims that psychological therapy is not the most effective way to change personality, but that being placed in a particular environment can produce greater changes in a shorter time. This gave rise to his experiments with milieu therapy, the creation of a total environment or therapeutic community, to achieve radical personality changes in those holocaust survivors who could not be reached by psychoanalysis.

138

Ben's quotation, earlier in this section, claimed a fundamental defining of self by being labelled and stigmatized as personality disordered. Ben went on to redefine the internal sense of self and external roles by taking up paid employment and, at a subsequent presentation about achievements, told the audience the following:

Ben: Although there are still good days and bad days, if you learn to love yourself you can begin to help others.

Recovery and maintaining healthy attachment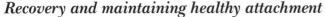

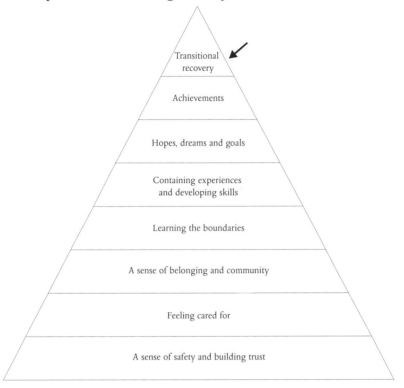

Figure 6.8 The pyramid of recovery: Transitional recovery.

Liberman and Kopelowicz (2005) have provided an operational definition of *recovery* and they discuss its outcomes. They make a distinction between *recovery* and *recovering* and show that it is not easy to separate the process from the outcome. Repper and Perkins (2003) speak of recovery being a process rather than a goal and represent it as a journey of recovery. Davidson (2003), within his definition of recovery, makes a distinction between living well with the illness and living beyond the illness. This concept suggests that the journey of recovery requires that the person does something rather than having something done to him or her by others. Such constructs are consistent with the last finding in our study. *Transitional recovery* emerged as both a concept and a vehicle. It embraced all other findings in that clients could continue their journey of recovery by defining and pursuing their unique goals and dreams, whilst still having a choice about whether to remain registered at The Haven or not.

Transitional recovery provides a new construct for personality disorder, with important implications for practice. It re-enforces The Haven ethos of reward for progress, rather than a response to illness and dysfunction which characterizes mainstream services. Related to the construct of recovery as a journey of small steps, namely a process rather than a goal, the concept of transitional recovery also addresses the issue of attachment. In psychological terms, healthy attachment ideally becomes internalized (Bowlby 1969). However, for those of us who have been lucky enough to have grown up with a safe base, this does not necessarily disappear in a material sense in adulthood. We are still able, in many cases, to have our families in our lives. If we have developed healthy attachment in our earlier years we are not hampered by difficulties in relating to others as we grow up. We have been able to form relationships and build networks anew. This is often not true for someone with a personality disorder diagnosis. At The Haven, if a healthy attachment had been formed, the concept of transitional recovery meant it would not be taken away:

Charles: I don't think we should clip our wings; we just need a nest to come back to.

The concept of transitional recovery was cited by participants as an approach that offered the layers of the pyramid and a safety net when required, and they acknowledged this need for intermittent support:

Leska: I personally think recovery is still being able to ask for support and say you are struggling but also know that you are getting better and that you don't need the services as much as you did when you were ill.

Participants feared losing their base and sense of home if they recovered. Because many had not developed a safe base in life they had no family or wider network of support to turn to if necessary. Some had achieved this at The Haven for the first time in their lives. Because the word recovery could potentially become synonymous with withdrawal of crucial support, it became vital to define what came next in a way that was going to be effective. Historically, recovery for people with mental health difficulties has followed a sequential path of treatment, recovery and rehabilitation. Transitional recovery offers a new way of working with people who have a personality disorder diagnosis. The pyramid of the journey of recovery in personality disorder addressed attachment issues, offered optional treatment, fostered hope and the regaining of control, and was embraced by the concept of transitional recovery where people could choose to retain a haven in which they might continue to develop and progress on their chosen path in the wider world:

Natasha: I have freedom to do what you want without being stopped by disability, getting on with your life in a productive way.

The original concept of capacity at the service was 100 to 110 clients. By the end of our study The Haven had registered 166 clients. It became possible to continue to accept new people because the choice of existing clients to remain at The Haven was contingent on using the service less, allowing new people to be registered at the project:

Sheila: I'm able to stand on my own two feet, without calling for help every five minutes.

The vehicle of implementing transitional recovery became the social inclusion unit at the service, where clients were able to work specifically on personal development skills related to their aspirations and achievements outside of The Haven. The development of this part of the service is described in the next chapter. Participants who had embraced the concept and structures of transitional recovery began to use The Haven less, while remaining registered at the service.

141

The Haven emerged as a unique model where therapeutic community principles were combined with those of a crisis house and the 24/7 nature of the service was cited by participants as a vitally important dimension. Therapies and services which exist for people with a diagnosis of personality disorder often require that the person meets certain criteria which represent readiness to work therapeutically. However, The Haven was able to hold and support many clients who did not yet meet such criteria. The re-creation of healthy attachment was combined with the principles of recovery, defined rather as *recovering*, representing a journey consisting of small steps. The entire structure of the service at The Haven was suggested and refined by its service users. Their unique knowledge about what would best support them and help them to progress shows that it is possible to work effectively with a relatively large number of people with a personality disorder diagnosis, well in excess of 100 at one time, many of whom had not made progress in other service settings, resulting in significant financial savings to the health, social care and the criminal justice system, see Appendix IX.

Boris: Though the past has not left me and there are a number of issues I still have to address, I am starting to get the life I now want, the life I have dreamed of since I was little. I am not doing what others ask of me I am following my dreams and my dreams alone. I now attend college and am currently seeking employment. I feel that I have lots to give and would be able to manage a job as well as my illness and I will still seek the support from the transitional recovery group if I ever have a difficult patch and need some help or guidance.

CHAPTER 7

A Journey of Organizational Change

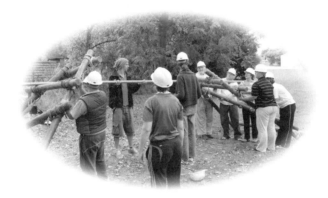

The Haven is consistent, it's been progressive and forward thinking, which is not a stale thing. It's not just something you go back to. It's something you go forward with. Anyone who tries to hold you back, they'll either be back at the hospital, or back in the situation they were before. If you hang on to The Haven you go forward.

Service User Quotation

What are the elements that constitute a *learning organization* and how does a participatory action research approach impact on organizational change? Here the process of *change* is related to the collective action-research nature of our research study and the increasingly participatory nature of stakeholder involvement.

The nature of The Haven

The Haven was a service which was created with some distinctly new and different features. It espoused aspects of the therapeutic community model where members would come together to explore emotional and psychological issues and exercise their decision-making and personal responsibility, while taking advantage of peer accountability. The setting for such organizations is usually residential and not based in the geographic area of participants, meaning they would take up residence at a service elsewhere in the country for a period of time (Hinshelwood 1999; Warren and Dolan 2001). Although the original concept of the therapeutic community suggested a retreat, over time the ethos of such communities embraced different models, some created as therapeutic community day units where participants could attend the program whilst retaining links to their home area (Rawlinson 1999). In the 1990s, crisis houses began to appear in different parts of the United Kingdom, offering short respite at difficult times. Not specializing in personality disorder, they were represented as a kind of asylum in the community, an alternative to psychiatric hospital (Tomlinson and Carrier 1996). Faulkner *et al.* (2002) championed the efficacy of the crisis house model, highlighting the user-led nature of such services and the emphasis on human interaction rather than drug treatments. Uniquely, The Haven was created as a blend of models combining a therapeutic community with a crisis house element. Therefore, participants could remain in their own geographic area, but also have the benefit of a short stay residential component within the service.

The concept of The Haven began essentially as a dissolution of earlier models and responses to care and treatment for personality disorder in our area. It sprang from a shared vision and creativity which, from the outset, aimed to be proactive and responsive to lessons and the need for change. This was not a service model imposed on an area but one coming out of previous user involved research (Ramon *et al.* 2001; Castillo 2003). It arose in a climate where pilot services for personality disorder were being proposed nationally by the Department of Health. As a daring response to the disappointment of previous service models, we were given carte blanche and, if our proposals for a service were agreed upon, we would receive the funding to pursue a pilot to test and develop our ideas for the care and treatment of personality disorder.

Learning organizations

Kofman and Senge (2001) speak of learning organizations being an exercise in personal commitment and community building. They suggest that this type of organization requires a re-definition of leadership to *servant leaders*. Such leaders are those who are walking ahead, and this is not necessarily dependent on management hierarchy. They propose that such leadership is intrinsically collective. Waiting for a leader to decide the way forward is a surrender of the power necessary to create a learning organization. This does not necessarily preclude management positions such as Chief Executive but, in order to reconcile potential dilemmas for learning organizations, this requires a value system that embraces leadership as a decision to serve. Servant leaders choose to serve one another and a higher purpose; a higher purpose such as helping each other to excel and achieve personal transformation.

On completion of our first research study (Castillo 2003) the service users involved in our journey found themselves, in the early 2000s, aggrieved and offended at the notion of untreatability in relation to personality disorder. From this sprang the hope for recovery. An important factor was the convergence of climates which existed in the new millennium. Not only was there a national focus on finding new ways forward for the support and treatment of personality disorder, the concept of *recovery* had also emerged in the mental health arena. This concept was led by service users in the USA, the UK, Australia, New Zealand and other countries. The first seeds for The Haven were sown during the initial research study conducted in the late 1990s, the emancipatory study carried out with service users who had a diagnosis of personality disorder. These seeds were nurtured during discussions with service users, from 2001 to 2003. The hope for recovery underpinned our efforts. In the planning of the service due consideration was given to evidence based treatments which already existed, especially therapeutic community models, which had an inherent flattened hierarchy, allowing staff and service users to 'walk ahead' together, as servant leaders.

The structure of The Haven

A revisiting of the structure of The Haven includes the crucial importance of the service being planned around the views and needs of the service users with the diagnosis. A proposal emerged which incorporated both a

24/7 crisis service and a therapies service with a tiered approach to group support and one-to-one work. The Haven Community Advisory Group was formed, with a democratically elected leader and deputy from amongst the client group. The acceptable behaviour policy was formulated with the clients and was administered by them. From the outset, structures were created that would allow service users to continue to drive developments at the service. Structures also ensured that clients would watch over and control behaviour, ensuring that the culture of the community would not be eroded, thereby instigating an ongoing learning process about self and others. Clinical matters were negotiated on an individual basis, between clients and staff, and confidentiality was preserved to the degree that the client would wish. That is, unless someone decided to share their personal, emotional and psychological matters with their peers, at groups or in community discussion, those matters would be entrusted only to the staff team. However, the shape of the services within The Haven, their efficacy, ideas for new developments, and many other matters regarding the day to day running of the service were client-led. For example, during a visit by three clients from another personality disorder service elsewhere in the country, we discovered that they had wanted a greenhouse in their grounds but had not been allowed to have one because this was deemed to be a self-harm risk. They also had a desire to hang pictures on their walls and to make their centre warm, welcoming and homely. They expressed their admiration for The Haven and compared the shortfalls in their own service. Many rules and policies were imposed from the top–down in their area, whereas The Haven's bottom–up approach gave the clients the decision about whether we should have a greenhouse in the garden, which we did, and about painting and decoration at the service. Our visitors said that when they asked about pictures they had been told that Blu Tack could not be used as it was damaging and picture hooks were a suicide risk as people could hang themselves. These types of decisions, which fundamentally characterize the atmosphere of an organization and its environment, were made by clients at The Haven.

Cycles of change

Action research is closely bound to practical action in an organization or social context. Main (1967) developed principles for a therapeutic organization which included the aspiration that 'the State of the organization is kept under continual examination and renewal'. This presents an organization as a learning system. Organizational learning is about the capacity and processes within an organization which can be used to improve performance (Nevis, DiBella and Gould 1995). Learning does not always occur in a linear way and can take place formally, informally and in unplanned ways. Checkland (1999) discovered that management education occurred, to a large degree, by making mistakes and watching others. In the development of his soft systems methodology he examined the non-linear, complex networks of interrelationships and interdependence, within organizational elements, which produce negative and positive feedback. Checkland concluded that organizational systems should be viewed in a systemic rather than a systematic way. A soft systems approach will encompass many perspectives of perceived reality, making comparisons of the whole in order to learn. Senge (1990, p.3) characterizes learning organizations as places where:

> *People continually expand their capacity to create the results they truly desire, where new and expansive patterns of thinking are nurtured, where collective aspiration is set free, and where people are actually learning to see the whole together.*

The participatory action research nature of our endeavour proved itself to be a vehicle for learning, creation and change. One of the main vehicles which created a feedback loop at The Haven was our research study and, as a result of issues raised by participants at the various research events, a series of changes were put into operation.

Implementing change

An array of potential stakeholders existed in relation to the creation of the service at The Haven, including policy makers, commissioners, external mental health professionals and the general public. The wishes of various stakeholders were likely to be different, for example, ranging from cost-savings achieved by a reduction in psychiatric hospital admissions to fewer disturbances from the range of symptomatology employed as coping strategies by clients with this diagnosis. However, the internal stakeholders involved in our journey of organizational change were the service users and the staff at The Haven. A transparency about information and the dialogue that had been set up with our clients was essential, and transcripts of research events with clients were made available to the staff. The clients' monthly Community Advisory Group was also attended by staff and minutes distributed widely, meaning that clients and staff not present at the meetings would be made aware of the dialogue and the issues. Similarly, minutes of all community discussions regarding unacceptable behaviour were distributed. Others closely associated, such as The Haven Board, included a number of service users in their membership and all were apparently in accord with how the service had been set up in relation to its recovery ethos, and the fact that it would encompass a bottom-up structure where clients were able to drive developments.

Nevertheless, although the staff team was committed to being responsive to the decisions of clients, this was a new and radical way of working for most of them. Also, recovery has a number of different meanings and, for many clients coming to this new service, it initially meant the right kind of support at critical times. During the planning of the service the high level of use of the crisis telephone line was underestimated. Participants soon made it clear, at the first research events in the study in February and May 2005 that the tension between support for crises in the building and crisis telephone use from outside the building was impacting detrimentally:

148

Collie: I was supposed to get a support call and it didn't come at all yesterday and I've got no answer to why it didn't come. I just thought that I ain't worth nothing. It feels like I don't belong here. (Service Evaluation Group May 05)

It was difficult for staff to hear such criticisms, especially as they were coming to grips with running a crisis service in a hectic climate and were, consequently, working very hard. It would have been easy to decide that the staff can't do everything; this client group is endlessly needy; they are projecting their earlier unmet needs onto the staff; and so forth. However, client comments were taken very seriously and it was decided that there was indeed a flaw in the system and, during the Spring of 2005, a new phone system was installed where, in addition to the mobile number for sending texts, the new system was given a dedicated crisis number, with a message saying that calls, if not answered immediately, should be responded to within 30 minutes. Additionally, short-term care plans began to include support calls, booked in the diary. The care plan forms were also created with a checklist on the back where staff could double check that all entries had been made in the diary before the plan was signed off, ensuring calls were not missed and opportunities for clients to feel rejected were reduced.

Setting up the new service had been a monumental effort in itself and no initial structures were created to include family members and carers. Therefore, a crucial group of stakeholders had been excluded. Clients began to call for *support for carers* during the first research event in February 2005:

Harry: I'd like to see something for carers. Carers get forgotten and services don't really help carers at all and, quite often, when they attend CPAs, and things like that, they're totally ignored. (Service Evaluation Group Feb 05)

In response, a Psycho-Educational Workshop was held at The Haven in September 2005, run by Kingsley Norton from the Henderson Hospital. Here, clients were able to bring their family members and carers for an afternoon of sharing problems and solutions. However, ongoing support for carers and family members was still not created at the service and again, this was called for by clients at the research event held in May 2006. The clients at The Haven research group also considered it was vital that some of the research focus groups should include family members and carers, and that research questions should also be included that would ask them about the kind of support they would like. The carer focus groups were held in March and August 2007. Here, our participatory action research process had led to a change in the research design itself and, as a result, family members and carers were enabled to express their views and ideas about what recovery meant for them and those they supported. Participants at those groups valued the support they gained from each other. In fact, during the first focus group it proved very difficult for the facilitator to keep the carers and family members to the agenda. There appeared to be so much pent up emotion on their part, and so much they wished to say, suggesting that their need for support was observably long overdue:

Alex: The chats that we have as carers, I think we can learn a lot from each other because we are discussing something with somebody else who knows where you are coming from and that just makes a difference. It's good for us all to see a different side isn't it? (Carers Focus Group March 07)

Sammy: I would like to see some kind of informal Carers Group run through The Haven. (Carers Focus Group Aug 07)

149

In response, a Family and Carers Group was established and held at The Haven each month.

Research feedback provided a high percentage of positive responses about what worked at the service and this is outlined in detail in Chapter 5 and in the appendices. Adopting a philosophy of 'if it ain't broke don't fix it', we kept doing what was working. However, the concept of *outreach* work became a frequent theme at service evaluation groups, client focus groups and interviews throughout the course of the research. As the initial needs of clients began to be met, in terms of crisis work and therapy, the need for outreach in the community was expressed. This included the desire for a range of help, from support in the home to support with children or in attending college:

Elise: There's an awful lot going on here in this building and on a one-to-one basis with clients, but there's nothing that I'm aware of that happens outside in the community. I really feel that one of the ways that recovery can be supported is if people are actually helping you to live lives in the actual community, outside of the four walls that are The Haven, helping people maybe have new flat starts and that kind of thing. (Service Evaluation Group Aug 05)

Jonny: Support on public transport as well, because I don't have a problem with it at all, but I know people do. (Service Evaluation Group Nov 05)

Poppy: I do feel I need outreach work for when I'm at home. (Client Focus Group Aug 06)

Fred: I need a little bit of help with moving. (Individual Interview April 07)

Leska: I have had a baby and I am feeling quite isolated and it's so hard to kind of still stay positive when you haven't got the support that helps you along with that and keeps you afloat. (Individual Interview July 07)

This presented itself as a particularly challenging feedback because the staff team was already stretched in their efforts to maintain successful actions in crisis and therapeutic work. As a way of addressing this need, student social workers were introduced to the service in September 2005 and, each year thereafter, a minimum of two students came on placement to The Haven:

Daniel: I think an important thing we do need to do is invite more student workers that are coming up to the finishing of their courses, to educate them in the mental health side, and not just letting them do the course and then letting their peers turn around to them and saying this is the way it should be done. (Service Evaluation Group Nov 05)

Students were also used for a range of outreach work, including supporting parents in the home:

Leska: One of The Haven social work students comes out most weeks to give us support and comes to any meetings I have. Because of this I don't feel secluded and I can still be part of The Haven. It's really nice to have someone to talk to, even if she is a chatterbox! But that's good distraction too. This has given me real practical and emotional support and I'm very grateful. (Individual Interview July 07)

Using students to help with core services within The Haven enabled both staff and students to become engaged in outreach work to help clients move home, attend meetings at college, negotiate public transport, and practise life skills such as shopping and looking after themselves in the home:

Natasha: Self-esteem and confidence, it's quite a major issue. I am getting some one-to-one support in going to college; someone's going to college with me. Going to college is quite a big deal. (Client Focus Group Nov 06)

Outreach statistics began to be kept in 2006 where they were averaging 20 hours a month. They eventually averaged 40 hours a month and outreach became a consistent part of the service provided at The Haven.

As the client base at the service grew new clients presented in crisis at the beginning of their journey. At service evaluation groups and client focus groups, participants highlighted the fact that they were aware of staff overload on crisis shifts, because of the need to respond to the many crises being presented by clients:

Christine: I think the staff sometimes cut themselves into lots and lots of pieces but I actually phoned in early in the morning, and my brain was telling me to do one thing and I thought I'll phone up and speak to somebody and unfortunately the staff were probably busy dealing with somebody else and it was too late when they did find me. When they rang me, the situation had happened. But I don't think it's an easy thing to overcome. I just don't think that the staff even carrying the phone around with them can be everywhere at once. I don't know how we can get around it. (Service Evaluation Group Nov 05)

This issue concurred with feedback from staff, therefore, by September 2006, in addition to the compliment of social work students which were added to the team, this situation was addressed by the introduction of volunteers to help with specific shifts where crisis contacts were proving most prolific.

Positive feedback also concerned therapies and group work. Early in 2005, as evidence-based therapy, the DBT skills group (dialectical behaviour therapy) was introduced to the group program. This was a structured group, requiring good commitment to sessions, and not all clients were ready or able to access the DBT skills program. However, participants felt it was important to learn life skills that would help them to understand and control their anxieties, and they began to express this need at research events during 2005:

Abigail: I don't know whether it's possible within the budget, the groups we have so far are very good, but I think anxiety management and I noticed you'd put a note on the board about anger management. Personally, anxiety management, if there was a group to do that I would appreciate it. (Service Evaluation Group Aug 05)

In 2005 the life skills program was developed. It ran weekly to encompass anxiety management, anger management, assertiveness and confidence building and addressed common difficulties associated with personality disorder such as self-harm, eating distress and substance misuse. The program was appreciated, however, help with such skills continued to be called for at research events during 2006:

Elise: The program of activities that runs needs to be constantly developed towards developing life skills for people so that, at the end of the day, they can actually go out and live that life. (Individual Interview Oct 06)

In response to this, by 2007 the life skills program had been expanded to include 18 weeks of sessions, encompassing managing finances, managing time and routines, sleeping difficulties and WRAP sessions (wellness recovery action plan). This continued as a rolling program of sessions that began again once the course was completed.

Short-term care plans were introduced soon after the service opened, as a proactive response to crisis support and care planning. This was an effort to work preventatively with clients by pre-booking support calls and one-to-one work each week. During the service evaluation groups and client focus groups in 2005, participants began to talk about the need to be supported to plan and look ahead:

Cosmic: I spent so many years just trying to get through the day that I've never actually had any long term plans. I wouldn't know how to start. (Service Evaluation Group Nov 05)

Some also spoke of being caught in a comfort zone. Staff responded by agreeing that they did not want to collude with that comfort zone and concluded that we needed to work with clients in a more in-depth way, looking at longer term issues and what would help each individual to move forward:

Jonny: Well that's going from short-term care plans to long-term care plans, isn't it? (Service Evaluation Group Feb 06)

Long-term care plans began to be introduced and, by 2006, a weekly clinical meeting was formed, called 'progress planning', where staff would discuss one or more clients each week, in a more in-depth way. Preliminary ideas for the long-term care plan were formulated at the meeting and taken to the client, to enable staff member and client to work on the plan together. In later years, at the suggestion of clients at the monthly advisory group meeting, many of whom felt the word 'care' felt medicalized, short-term care plans were renamed support plans and long-term care plans became lifeplans. Eventually, the feedback loop came full circle in that an annual review, or re-registration, took place for each client who wished to remain registered at the service. Here, a section of the annual review form included the pyramid of our journey of recovery in personality disorder, where clients were given time to reflect on their progress on the pyramid and to see, from their own individual perspective, how the layers related to each other, and to pinpoint where they might have become stuck and where they were progressing. The annual review form ended with a lifeplan or an update of that person's lifeplan if one already existed.

It is difficult to evaluate whether some of the changes described above would have occurred despite the research. I would argue that they occurred substantially because of it, due to the feedback loop established by the ongoing dialogue that had been opened with clients. One change that did occur was not connected directly to research feedback. It was, however, related to the proactive ethos adopted at the service in terms of care planning and a preventative approach. This concerned the use of the crisis beds. Initially, four beds existed at the service and a stay would be anything from one night up to three weeks.

Nomenclature was an important factor here because the term 'crisis bed' suggested that someone had to be in crisis to obtain one. This had the potential to provoke a competition of crises to see who might be most deserving of a bed. It was also noted by staff that, in our early days, clients would not infrequently overdose on discharge from a crisis bed stay. This occurred despite the 24/7 nature of the service, which was geared for contact on discharge from a bed and which would even ensure transport to the service at critical times of the day or night. Thought and discussion from the staff team yielded ideas about using the four beds in a different way. These changes were taken to the client group and agreed with them. Respite stays began to be planned ahead. They were contingent on good engagement. It was also important to agree with clients whether the bed stay had been beneficial. One of the ways formulated to do this was to see how that client coped in the week after discharge from a bed before agreeing the booking for their next respite bed stay. Subsequent to the introduction of this decision, or cunning plan, the number of overdoses after discharge from a bed miraculously plummeted. Although there were times when a client was admitted to a bed at The Haven when they were in crisis, especially to avoid a psychiatric hospital admission, the majority of bed stays became pre-booked as respite stays, for example, a week every two months or two weeks every three months. This proved to be a way to encourage progress and to give clients the hope of planned respite to enable them to manage their recovery. Clients used beds in different ways. Some booked a stay during difficult anniversaries, others planned challenging therapeutic work during a stay to ensure they would be safe during that time, others used the stay as a kind of holiday and a break from day to day pressures.

A need for change which clients found hard to articulate ——

Concurrent with service users' lessons regarding *boundaries*, The Haven staff team was also engaged in its own process of learning the boundaries and it is essential that our hard-won lessons regarding this issue are included here. Gutheil and Gabbard (1993), who are international experts in the field of boundaries in clinical practice, suggest that both complex and lesser boundaries pose significant challenges for clinicians. Sometimes clearly delineated but often amorphous, certainly at the outset, the response to boundary issues for the staff team required not just the creation of clear policy, but also the espousing of openness and systems where staff could share and receive peer perspectives.

Because they have often experienced early traumatic events, and overwhelmingly unmet needs in early and later life, people diagnosed with personality disorder may have little sense of boundaries (Mahari 2004). An individual needs to have a sense of their own identity and space, and the identity and space of another, in order to have an awareness of boundaries. Someone with a personality disorder diagnosis may not be aware of where they end and you begin. Demands placed on professionals and others can be experienced by them as a violation of boundaries and limits and may cause a mental health worker to either become over involved or to distance themselves from someone with this diagnosis.

Hinshelwood (1998) suggests that difficult patients create reactions in those who try to care for and treat them. Kerr (2001) speaks about the idea of 'the ailment as ignorance', that is, a lack of understanding may cause others to respond either by becoming too closely associated with a client, or by regarding that individual as too difficult a patient to work with. Both approaches further affect that person's mental health in an adverse way. He explains that behaviour is also a form of communication and that the way in which a system responds to this behaviour may also be dysfunctional. He urges us to see things in a *systemic* way, as a series of dynamics being enacted around that person. Services and people around the client may be reacting in a variety of ways, identifying, sympathizing and becoming inappropriately involved, or getting angry with and rejecting the client, feeling guilty or burnt out, a variety of responses which fall short of actually understanding how it is for that individual. This can be experienced as a minefield which presents a significant challenge to any staff team who may be subject to extreme boundary testing. Confronted with a therapeutic community environment such as The Haven, staff and clients co-existing

155

in a close atmosphere are sometimes exposed to a hazardous excess of emotions. For this reason boundaries must be negotiated, drawn, and clearly understood by clients and staff alike. Boundaries must be consistent and allow clients to take stock of thoughts and feelings and learn to take responsibility for how their actions impact on themselves and others, and staff must understand clearly how this works.

In the early years at the service, personnel difficulties were experienced in terms of boundary breaking. It is not possible to discuss the details of these issues here. They were also not disclosed in any research event, including individual client interviews. Staff felt the need to discuss the boundary issues with certain clients who had been affected but were reticent to do so because they felt clients should not be burdened and involved. This, however, presented a deadlocked situation with insufficient information because the alleged boundary issues were denied by the staff members concerned. The Vulnerable Adults Lead from the local Mental Health Trust was consulted and pointed out that many in this client group were used to keeping secrets within the family and it would be a great disservice not to help them bring matters out into the open because, by not doing so, we could be replicating patterns of early abuse. We were urged to at least give the clients involved an opportunity to do so. The acceptable behaviour policy for clients at the project had been written at the outset. Now, as a result of the information service users disclosed about staff boundary violations, it became necessary to create policies for staff which spelled out and made boundaries very explicit.

Retaining humanity, while holding firm boundaries, sometimes requires flexibility and can leave grey areas that will always exist with this client group. Opportunities at staff meetings, individual supervision and teambuilding needed to be safe enough, and to occur often enough, for a culture of openness to thrive. If someone is drawn into a compelling situation it can be much easier for colleagues to see what is happening. Our procedure at The Haven was to bring all issues to the staff team, bring them to supervision, write them in client notes, and discuss them openly and in an authentic way with the client. Boundary issues were always up-for-debate at The Haven. The occasions that we ran into difficulties were the times when issues became hidden. Professionals may enter the mental health field because they have a history of psychological difficulties and are trying to understand or overcome their own problems. This is the concept of the 'wounded healer' where someone is compelled to treat or care for another because they are 'wounded' themselves (Jung 1954). The professional may or may not be consciously aware of his or her own personal wounds. These wounds may be activated in certain situations especially if the wounds are similar. Key learning at The Haven included the fact that where a staff member had unresolved personal difficulties, and un-drawn boundaries, working with this client group could become untenable. Working with personality disorder is not for everyone and requires a truly honest and fairly constant examination of working practices for a staff member, and support systems that allow that person to do so (Castillo 2009).

During the national evaluation of the 11 community personality disorder pilots, of which The Haven was one, part of the study concerned burnout rates for staff (Crawford *et al.* 2010). The study cited prevalence of aggression and suicidal behaviour as high risk factors for staff burnout, and noted that such behaviours are common amongst those with a personality disorder diagnosis. However, the study found that burnout rates were lower amongst the staff groups at the national personality disorder pilots. The recruitment of reflective and resilient personnel, an emphasis on teamwork and mutual support and reflective practice involving forums where staff could regularly come together, were all factors which were highlighted as reducing work-related anxiety and burnout. Many staff involved in the study emphasized the positive aspects of working with this client group and reported a sense of achievement in their work.

After six years of operation and subsequent to our many hard-won lessons, at a Haven teambuilding meeting 2010, staff discussed the recently published national evaluation (Crawford *et al.* 2010) and added their thoughts. Some talked of the team being the best they had ever worked with. They valued team interdependence and the fact that colleagues looked after each other. They discussed how support was enhanced in service structures from handovers, to teambuilding, to clinical supervision. Some spoke of their commitment to working with this client group because they had struggled to support them in other service settings. Many staff spoke of The Haven as a unique service and said that they felt part of something challenging and different and believed that there was both a sense of freedom to be oneself but also firm structures and boundaries. Some staff spoke of not being drained at work for the first time ever and about feeling glad to walk through the door to work. Mirroring the views of clients, some spoke of it being a safe place to work with a sense of belonging and being part of a family. One said, 'It's like coming home.'

Rewarding positive progress

Although research feedback about the services provided continued to indicate that they were successful and supportive, some participants, in the privacy of individual interviews rather than focus groups, began to make powerful statements about recovery and the importance of *rewarding positive progress*:

Elise: I think, fundamentally, people with PD need a certain amount of love and care and TLC and pampering and I think The Haven's taken that well on board and has supplied that, where other statutory units have failed dismally. I do think it's very easy to pour out the love and concern and that's so important because so many people haven't had that, but then I think there's a danger that that then becomes an emotional crutch and people don't particularly want to move on. That dependency shouldn't be fostered; it should be actively discouraged in a very gentle way. (Individual Interview Oct 06)

Cosmic: The staff could be more accessible and stop spending all their time on attention seekers and people that just go home, get wrecked and come back, and are on that cycle. (Individual Interview Nov 06)

However, others spoke of the need for continued healthy attachment and support:

Pablo: I'm not a blubbering wreck in the corner. I've got specific times when I can't cope. But I've learnt to stop, yeah, I come here. I literally come in and sit down. It stops the ball rolling, puts a wedge under the ball. It works and keeps me in the right space that keeps my clarity, keeps my sobriety right. (Individual Interview Aug 06)

The concept of transitional recovery was adopted in late 2006 in an effort to address both needs expressed above, by allowing clients to stay registered at The Haven as a safety net whilst making positive progress. The Haven had been planned primarily around its service users' views and ideas. They had asked for a 24-hour crisis service, and this had been refined over time in accordance with their views. Similarly, therapy services had been set up in accordance with clients' ideas, providing one-to-one support and group work. This part of the service was also refined over time in response to views and ideas expressed at research events. The concept of transitional recovery and the desire for social inclusion were not something envisioned by clients during their original planning of the service. The degree of crises and the need for care, support and therapeutic work obscured the arena of the outside world. One of the first accessories acquired at the service, in 2004, was a board for 'Blue Sky Thinking' where clients could take a white dove and write on it their dream for recovery and then pin it on the board. What was written on the doves was humbling and included needs such as, *'Just to be listened to'; 'Someone to understand'; 'I just want to feel safe'*. Two years later, although the need for support and care was still apparent, a different kind of need began to be expressed:

Harry: For those that are further along in their recovery, interview techniques would be handy, to help get there, practise role play and get them used to the process with college and employment. (Service Evaluation Group May 06)

Rose: My goal is to go to university to get my MA and then take it further. (Service Evaluation Group May 06)

Tiffany: The Haven should help us get voluntary work. (Client Focus Group Nov 06)

Jenny: I now want to do my access course and I want to work in care. (Individual Interview Feb 07)

This heralded the most fundamental shift in the shape of Haven services. Now our participatory learning and change process led to proposing role transition. By the end of 2006 a transitional recovery group began to be held weekly in an effort to support clients to work towards such goals. Once clients at the service realized that they would not lose The Haven if they made progress, over half of the client group signed up to transitional recovery. We began a group which was packed with attendees each week. One staff member had some 11-plus school mathematics exam papers which she brought to the group during our early weekly sessions. We all set out to fill in the papers, staff and clients alike. At one stage I looked up across the room in amazement at all the heads bowed over papers and pens scribbling industriously, and I thought to myself that to be spending the afternoon doing something like an arithmetic exam surely proved that so many of our clients truly wanted to progress.

Eight months later, in July 2007, we were able to open a social inclusion unit at The Haven with a full-time coordinator, teaching a range of personal development skills, and a part-time assistant to help her to support clients in fulfilling their hopes, dreams and goals in their journey of recovery. This was an organizational change, and fundamental augmentation of The Haven model that we had never envisioned at the outset. It had not been factored into our original funding proposal. The financing of the new unit came from Her Majesty's Cabinet Office Social Exclusion Task Force. The task force offered start-up funding only but we believed our successful efforts, in terms of maintained client stability and achievements in the outside world, would encourage local commissioners to take over the funding for this newer part of the service once the initial two years were complete. In a difficult financial climate, and despite a third year's funding from the Cabinet Office, local commissioners felt unable to fund the unit further. It was true that because the social inclusion unit was set up with temporary funding this made it more susceptible to rejection in the current economic climate, especially when medical rather than social interventions for mental health problems had traditionally received more investment.

However, local commissioners also seemed to be questioning the outcome measures cited by The Haven, even though the outcomes for the overall service showed very significant service and cost-savings and our systematic research endeavours additionally showed important changes in the quality of life of our clients. I continue to question the suitability of instruments, such as the Health of the Nation Outcome Scale (HoNOS), in terms of their ability to measure recovery, compared to the value of subjective instruments based on service user stories. Wallcraft (2011) advocates a bottom–up approach to the development of more sensitive measures, which will involve service users in their creation. Paid employment is often cited as the epitome of a professional notion of recovery. Fifteen per cent of Haven clients were at that time engaged in paid employment or permitted work, which was much higher than the national average of 3.4 per cent for people with mental health problems (Work, Recovery and Inclusion, HMSO 2009). We considered that we could measure-up to a variety of desirable outcomes. However, even though The Haven was engaged in a process of rewarding clients for positive progress, it seemed that the service itself would not in turn be rewarded for its positive progress.

The news about this decision came just three months before the Cabinet Office set-up funding was due to cease and we felt devastated.

Up to this time we had lived a charmed life. Now someone had said 'no'. During discussions with service users and other stakeholders, in the days after we had received the news, it became clear that there was a will to raise the funds necessary to continue and a determination not to lose this part of the service. The social inclusion unit at The Haven had emerged as a product of organizational learning and change and its stakeholders were not about to stand back and see it disappear. In the first week of 2010 the snow fell heavily and the buses were cancelled. However, many service users walked to The Haven in the snow. This continues to be a memory that moves me greatly. Their resolve to reach The Haven on that day was to attend a special meeting to plan what should be done. A campaign was launched and the servant leaders of the organization 'walked ahead'. Both staff and service users, together, took the lead on raising funds. This began with a media campaign:

Boris: It's about supporting someone through troubled times, encouraging them to college, giving something back; being part of a bigger picture, improving someone's quality of life, and feeling safe. (BBC TV Look East News – 10 January 2010)

Doris: The Haven has helped me to get on an even keel and addressed stuff that's happened in the past. Since the social inclusion unit started it's helped me realize the person I can be. I want to be the best (me) in the world. I had the devil on my back in the form of a Math's GCSE. It took me seven attempts and, last year, with the help of the Social Inclusion Department I finally obtained it. (Local Gazette – Vital Project's Funding Plea – 26 January (Calnan 2010))

Emily: By the time I was thirty-five I was an alcoholic. I was self-harming, having flash back of sexual abuse when I was a kid and I was suicidal. I was on life support about five times. Since I've been at The Haven I haven't been back in hospital for four years. I haven't had a drink in twenty-six months. With the support of the Social Inclusion Unit I have two NVQs for English and Volunteering. I now do voluntary work. (Local Gazette – Vital Project's Funding Plea – 26 January (Calnan 2010))

Lesley Allen, the first service user to make her views known in 1998, during our original research endeavour (Castillo and Allen 2003), was living out of the district during the time The Haven research took place. However, she now returned to the area to receive support from the Social Inclusion Unit at The Haven in seeking employment. In a full circle return to campaigning, Lesley took the lead in a letter which was sent out nationally:

Excerpt from Lesley's letter:

> Twelve years ago, in 1998, as a service user with this diagnosis I became part of the original campaign to highlight the plight of those with personality disorder and, from the efforts of service users with the diagnosis in North East Essex, I have seen The Haven come into being from a dream to an embryo, to being the current flourishing service. It is with real sadness that I write to confirm that, as some of you already know, funding has not been able to be agreed to continue The Haven's social inclusion unit. This is a vital part of our service and we are now trying to find alternative funds to retain two valued and knowledgeable members of staff and keep the other activities in the unit going. It seems ironic that, just as national guidance such as 'New Horizons' and 'Realizing Ambitions' is hot off the press, aiming for social inclusion and work opportunities for people with mental health problems, this is the very part of The Haven service that has come under threat. (27 January 2010)

Finally, one of our research participants wrote a testimonial and wished to have this circulated widely. It was sent out nationally, as part of Lesley's letter and is excerpted below:

Ben: I have personality disorder…in effect, a dustbin diagnosis that marked the end-of-the-line of hope for recovery. The success of the care is nothing short of astonishing. Over a period of time I have changed from an emotional cripple with no self-esteem and certainly no future in society, to a working professional, with a strong network of friends and a fully-functioning family. This situation was created in no small part with the full assistance of the social inclusion team at The Haven. Despite my years of self-loathing, this unit gave me every skill and confidence to fight my way back into society. And they remain there for me if I need their support again. (27 January 2010)

True to their word that the Social Inclusion Unit would not close, by June 2010 stakeholders had managed to secure most of the required £60,000 funding for the current financial year and remained resolved to continue to fundraise for the following financial year. Successful fundraising for the social inclusion unit continued over the following years.

I believe that this later development was an expansion of participatory action research in a true Frierian (1970) sense. The group as a whole was an agent for change in that it sought solutions that shaped their lives and, in doing so, it engaged a wider, often passive public. The Haven now became even more connected to the non-NHS world, through involving people from the media, and in reaching so many others who gave donations and became legitimate stakeholders of the service.

Outdoor well-being

Social exclusion can be exacerbated by the fact that the concept of the personality disorder diagnosis itself attracts stigma and discrimination (Social Exclusion Task Force 2006). When funding was obtained from Her Majesty's Cabinet Office Social Exclusion Task Force and the social inclusion unit at The Haven was opened, it enabled the employment of not only a dedicated coordinator and a part-time assistant, but also a part-time educational tutor and a parenting classes tutor. Plans continued to encompass all domains of social inclusion; income; housing; leisure; tackling stigma and discrimination; families and children; education; voluntary work and paid employment. Transitional recovery 'took wing'.

163

Important developments in confidence building also occurred as part of the work of the social inclusion unit at The Haven. In the late 1990s, while still working as a mental health advocate, I was asked by the local mental health trust to carry out a survey of in-patient services in the west of the county. Back then, we visited all the wards on site; acute psychiatric in-patient admissions; older people's wards; secure psychiatric provision. One thing we kept hearing was that a ward had once existed, by this time closed, a rehabilitation ward which had many patients who we felt had probably been diagnosed with personality disorder. This ward had instigated a program of outward-bound activities, taking service users on walking and climbing expeditions and engaging them in many other outdoor activities. We were told that a fair number of patients made significant progress in their journey of recovery and became completely discharged from mental health services. This piece of information was something that lodged in the back of my mind. Therefore, in 2007, when the new social inclusion coordinator suggested some activities outdoors I enthusiastically agreed. This began with visits to the Outdoor Centre on Mersea Island where Haven clients, of all ages, engaged in teambuilding activities and negotiating the assault course. The culmination of some of these wonderful days at the Outdoor Centre was to be brave enough to climb the tower and slide down the zip wire. Disabled clients, some even wheelchair-bound, negotiated this challenge with pride. During the next seven years Mersea Island offered other valuable pursuits in the form of bushcraft activities and care farming, collectively known as *Outdoor Well-being* (Castillo 2013).

Doris: A day here has helped me to ground myself and just be. The chickens don't care how you're feeling, they just want to be fed. I'm busy doing 'real' stuff, being reminded of the food-chain and our place in it. Being productive and feeling valued.

Brunhilda: Hopefully, it will also open up opportunities for future paid or voluntary work, to say nothing of the increased sense of well-being.

Outdoor well-being activities continued on a weekly basis in more recent years, broadening out a few miles into the countryside between the Blackwater Estuary and the River Colne, still encompassing Mersea Island and some other little bits of heaven situated in that area. Clients relating their journeys in the next chapter, speak about their experiences with the Outdoor Wellbeing Program.

Shared power and participatory action

Kofman and Senge (2001) propose that organizational learning is engendered by groups who espouse capabilities beyond the traditional: empathy, compassion, even love they would say, practices that generate conversation, dialogue and collaborative action, and which have the capacity to see work as a system which is a flow of life. The values of an organization are its life blood and service users as stakeholders were setting forth on a life journey that circumstances may have previously robbed them of, or perhaps never allowed them to develop. Such organizations necessarily attract staff and other stakeholders who have compassion and flexibility of thought. The Haven research initiative did not seek the views of its staff members during the course of the study; however, the way the organization adapted and changed suggests that, after some initial difficulties, the service mainly chose well in its staff team and other major stakeholders, such as its Board of Directors.

Recovery-led services require an adjustment at the power base of any organization and, at The Haven, the use of a participatory action research approach led to fruitful changes. A learning organization is a collective action (Kofman and Senge 2001) and requires a shift that changes the core of how we work. The Haven, as an organization, attempted to espouse such principles and became a living, learning and changing community.

CHAPTER 8

Four Journeys

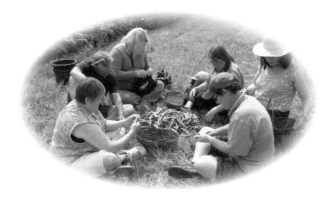

I have actually discovered life. It's not even a rediscovery. It's a discovery. Looking at how I am living now, I haven't lived up to now, I have just been surviving. I'm talking about success as in how happy and content you are as a person, success in life rather than qualifications and a good job. It's very individual for each of us. It's about breaking out of your own mould that you've made or other people have made for you. It's about breaking out of that mould.

Service User Quotation

Since completion of our second research study it was always our intention to augment findings with some updated and fuller stories, or case studies. The four following journeys: *Getting out; Include me in; Getting grounded; Moving on;* represent this augmentation. Our research study reflected the thoughts and experiences of 60 of our service users, and yielded many of their words. They were necessarily snapshots of experiences and learning which accumulated into realizations about the journey of recovery for people with a personality disorder diagnosis, which gave validity to our research and displayed the trustworthiness of our findings. The additional and fuller reports in this chapter were written in 2013 and are aimed to be qualitative accounts inviting the reader into the inner world of some of our participants.

Each of our four storytellers in this chapter has opened his or her heart, life and experiences with candour. These stories are not of the ordinary because they lie at the hinterland of human experience. They lead us into a world of fragmented mental processes, extreme emotions and mortal danger, not least from one's own hand, danger stemming from traumatic loss, and from inhumane treatment and institutions.

All registered clients were invited to tell their stories and the four included here were by self-selection. A fifth participant, who was the service user who led the focus groups and carried out the individual interviews in The Haven research study, also expressed the desire to write about this experience and her account follows the four journeys.

Getting out: by EJ

I was 15½ years old when I was first detained under the English Mental Health Act. Caught setting a fire in some shrub land, I was sent to a remand centre and before long I found myself in Ashworth, one of Britain's high security mental hospitals. Thirty-six years later I was still in hospital, yet the only charges I had ever faced were for arson after the fire in the shrub land, and one charge of theft.

My father was an army man. He was strict and a military man to the core. I was not really the son he would have wished for because, from an early age, I liked female things and I used to wear my sister's clothes. Then I stole some women's clothes from a washing line. I knew it was wrong but I felt compelled. One can only imagine the impact of these events on a man such as my father. He tried everything from boys' boarding school to boot camp at the army base. I was confused about my gender and identity, about my place in the family and my place in life. I felt alone and unloved. The land where I set the fire had belonged to the army and, in retrospect, I wonder if in setting light to it I was somehow trying to punish my father for my deep dilemma and whether this was an unconscious cry for help. The 'help' I received was not quite what I had bargained for.

In the 1970s the British Special Hospitals were a strange and alien land. Everything was highly regulated including our work regime which began early each morning with scrubbing the floors of the hospital from one end to the other. Then we polished them from one end to the other. When that was done we started at the beginning again. At one stage, after I had graduated to the woodwork section, I was making a chair and I asked whether this was work or therapy? I was told it was therapy. It was over 30 years before I met a psychologist.

Sometimes the staff actually caused patients to fight with each other and then they would write, 'Patient A attacked patient B for no reason'. There was always a reason. There was no privacy in terms of dressing and undressing and we were given cardboard toiletiers for our night waste and we had to carry these out for disposal in the morning. It was very degrading. I've even known patients to use human waste as a weapon; the last refuge of the disempowered. Many things were taken away from us, like photographs I had as keepsakes from my childhood. These were very personal memories from my past. I was lucky to begin with because I was allowed four visits a year. But my family stopped coming after a while. I think I was an embarrassment and they didn't know what to do about me.

During the time I was held in hospital under the Mental Health Act I had many chances to appeal against my detention. For some years I took advantage of the annual opportunity to have my case reviewed at a tribunal. On each occasion the tribunal panels recommended that I be transferred to a hospital of lesser security. As early as 1992, one mental health review tribunal stated, 'It is becoming something of a scandal that after all these years this patient is still in special hospital, particularly as it is probable that he has never been mentally ill at all.' This sentiment was repeated again and again in consecutive reviews. Eventually recommendations simply stated, 'Detention in maximum security is not necessary.'

In the mid-90s I was eventually transferred to Severalls Hospital, the local institution in Colchester. The next day I was sent on leave to town. I couldn't cope. The change was too great. I stole a car and got swiftly transferred back to Ashworth Special Hospital. My tribunal solicitor said, 'Part of the problem is that if you leave people in institutions too long they become institutionalized. It's like gate fever. They sort of get lost and abandoned in the system, and after a while they can't cope with life outside the hospital. With this particular case, I don't think he ever needed maximum security in the first place, but he got kind of stuck there. Now he is so institutionalized that he doesn't know anything else.' Over the years I was transferred to Rampton Special Hospital and the appeal tribunals continued. The Independent on Sunday newspaper covered my story and, although I wasn't able to speak to the newspaper directly, I was able to communicate through my solicitor.

After the newspaper article was published it took another five years for me to be discharged from hospital, but this was a Conditional Discharge. Therefore, I was still held under section of the Mental Health Act, but in 2007 I was moved to Colchester to a hospital in the community and registered at The Haven. The Haven has done me a lot of good and has given me a lot of confidence and support. I really feel part of the community here at The Haven. Because I lost touch with my family a long time ago I think of The Haven like a home and family. However, I was still being held under the Mental Health Act. My freedom was curtailed. I could go so far in life, but not as far as I wanted. What if I wanted to go on holiday or choose the accommodation I really wanted to live in? There was also a psychological sense of not being allowed to be myself. I had applied for so many appeal tribunals over the years and then, fantastically, on 19 November 2010, after 40 years of being held under a section of the Mental Health Act, I attended yet another tribunal and my section was LIFTED! I don't feel it was right to detain me for so long. There may have been concerns, but to restrict a human being for so long is a violation of human rights.

Part of my sense of freedom was to be able to dress the way I like. This is who I am and if people don't accept it that's up to them. I harm no-one. Once when I was working as a volunteer at the Oxfam Charity Shop a customer said, 'You look very nice today young lady,' with no malice aforethought, and said very pleasantly in fact. However, I more usually get stupid comments from members of the public, but you have to be strong. The Haven has always accepted me for who I am from day one. This makes me strong. Another freedom was to move into my own place. Some may say I have too many cats! I might have five, but I'm not saying. If you can't look after them don't have them. I look after mine well. I love and care for my cats and they all come running to me when I get home each evening.

With the support I now have I can carry on with my life and the challenges I meet. I have been invited to Anglia Ruskin University five times to speak to the students there and tell my story. I've made them laugh and I've made they cry. One group asked how I had managed to survive it all and I told them that each day I used to say to myself, 'One day at a time sweet Jesus'. I've also done a number of voluntary jobs, the last one being the Bicycle Initiative and they want me back next year. I was also a founder

169

member of the Outdoor Well-being Program at The Haven and one of the early 'guinea pigs' for Bushcraft, the Mersea Island Activities Centre, and for going down to the farm. You might have seen my photograph, hugging lambs or fishing, in some of our reports.

Ever since I gained my freedom I have had a dream about going back on a holiday to Hong Kong where I was born. I've been saving for a long time and I now have my passport. I am ready and I got a good travel deal. The hotel is booked. Kowloon here I come. I am going to take lots of photographs and when I get back I'll have a special session at the transitional recovery group at The Haven to give everyone a Hong Kong film show. I am getting a Hawaiian shirt so that when I go to the butterfly sanctuary the butterflies will land on me. And…best of all…I will see the magical Fire Dragon Dance.

In March 2014, EJ died of natural causes after a short illness. EJ did visit Hong Kong as planned, had a wonderful holiday and also presented a slide show of the visit to the Transitional Recovery Group. Despite 36 years of hospitalization, EJ's last seven years were spent in freedom and the pursuit of happiness. Even in death EJ remains an inspiration.

Include me in: by Joseph Brown

I don't want to talk about my early history here. Suffice to say I left home aged 15, a home that was, by any standards, a very abusive environment. Somehow I functioned until my 30s. I was a sportsman, a badminton champion, a dog trainer, and a father. All these parts of me were outside identities, but inside I was lost. Somehow I had blanked out that early history and I know other people who have done the same thing, only to break much later, spectacularly and unexpectedly.

Eventually my behaviour became erratic. I didn't understand what was happening. I experienced paranoia and the terrible fear that I was being followed. I assigned strange significances to things like the stars and to sounds. I was admitted to a psychiatric hospital. I stopped eating in order to starve myself to death. This turned into anorexia. When I started eating again I began to cut myself. No-one told me I had been diagnosed with a personality disorder. I was admitted to psychiatric hospital 36 times, mostly under section of the Mental Health Act, and I was also sent to specialist eating disorder clinics three times. Although I met some very caring professionals within psychiatric services, the experience left me without hope. What was my sense of identity? I don't think I could even conceive of having one at this time and I felt so hopeless I tried to set light to myself twice in hospital.

I met my wife during this time and she has been my carer and my godsend. She has loved me and looked after me through mental illness, cancer and disabling arthritis. I wonder whether I would be here today without her. Seven years ago I came to The Haven and the tide really began to turn for me. I have not been back in hospital and neither have I self-harmed since I have been at The Haven. It took me a long, long time to gain enough trust to be able to talk about my past, and I'm still talking, I'm getting there. But The Haven seems to understand the process of trust and the time it takes for some of us to feel safe enough when our formative experiences in life have been so excruciatingly unsafe. I've really used the groups at The Haven and learned the skills to help cope with my feelings and impulses.

This year I became brave and joined the transitional recovery group at The Haven. I avoided that group for quite some time because I thought that being 'recovered' would mean I would lose The Haven and I certainly didn't feel that would be right for me. But I didn't know what I was missing at that group. Then the idea of transitional recovery was properly explained to me and now I understand that it doesn't mean cure. I understand that this is my journey of recovery and my life and that it's a journey of little steps that just goes on and on. I finally understood that I wouldn't lose The Haven if I made progress in the journey. In fact I realized that this is what The Haven is all about.

So I joined the transitional recovery group and I am working with the social inclusion staff at The Haven on the weekly outdoor well-being program. It's been fantastic! I've been down on the farm, out in a boat, I've hugged hens, walked for miles with my crutches, I've flown a kite, I've been fishing, sat round the campfire, and learned compass and map reading. I love it so much. It's like I was on the outside of things but now I'm on the inside. Not only am I included in the group I'm included in life really.

I know that, as I have improved, my wife has begun to worry. It's been difficult for her and I know she has felt that I might not need her so much. But I need her so much just to be in my life and celebrate my progress and increasing independence. So we are both now in a phase of transition, or transitional recovery, and our relationship will change and grow as I grow.

My one great sadness is that, along the way, I lost my daughter. It could not have been easy for her, having a parent with such serious problems. I was so ill at one stage I even smashed up the house. I understand the impact this must have had on a child but I have wanted so much to be re-united with her. Last Christmas I took a chance and sent a Christmas card…then I received one back. I waited and waited for her to phone on Christmas day. She didn't phone. I picked up a drink for the first time in eight years. The cooking sherry! It was all that was in the house. I felt so guilty. In the New Year, at The Haven life skills group they saw the funny side of it, me drowning my sorrows with the cooking sherry. Other people at the group said I shouldn't give up. So I didn't give up but decided to simply step back and quietly hope.

To this day I have still not heard from my daughter. But this year The Haven had a summer fete and I sat in the back garden tending the bric-a-brac stall and looked over at a young man and his children and felt some sense of recognition. I found out later that he had asked one of the staff my name and said he thought I was his Granddad. Moments later I was speaking to my grandson and my three baby great-grandsons. What a Casablanca moment…of all the fetes in all the towns…the joy was indescribable, and completely unexpected, overwhelming, a piece of utter magic. Even staff members were in tears. So…include me in the family… include me in life…include me in, in, in.

Getting grounded: by Helen Price

I sat at my Mum's bedside, watching her die, willing her to live at any cost. I walked through the corridors alone, trying to be strong for all those who would be affected. Their pain was strong, but eventually it evaporated. Maybe I don't want the grief of Mum's death to leave, because if I do, then it would be like letting her go. Even the heartache it causes is better than thinking for a moment that I have forgotten her. I thought I knew 'death'. I was sure I had a handle on what to do, and how to feel. I look back at Dad's death with a detached feeling. I was too little to understand. Dogs lasted longer than Dads in my world. With Dad there was anger and frustration, but how much of that was down to a little person trying, unsuccessfully, to comprehend terms like 'suicide' 'funeral ' and 'inquest'. I guess I never really mourned my loss. It got quickly swept up in ballet shoes, and famous fives… I wanted to be as little bother to Mum as possible. As a small person, I couldn't make it all better, or make the horror of finding your husband, swinging, go away. But I could be as good as I could be.

If my personality describes 'who I am' then what gives anyone the right to describe it as 'disordered'. Because that would insinuate that I am disordered…that there's something wrong or bad inside me, a fundamental flaw in my make-up, which confirms what I have always thought; I am 'bad', even though I have always tried to be good; I'm dysfunctional. I have endured patronizing doctors, nosey counsellors and interfering nurses. They all appear to be pre-programmed to dismiss my self-loathing, while at the same time confirming it with a diagnosis, given to me by them, that highlights my 'disordered' sense of self. I am more than a label, as we all are…but once identification with this label has been made, everything one ever was is dismissed. All that made you you is erased, all your previous morals, studies, discoveries and achievements gone.

To the untrained eye, and on a good day, I can appear as though I haven't a care in the world. I can socialize, use public transport, walk for miles, cook and do my washing. To get this far has taken years, years to be built back up, periodically returning to maladaptive coping mechanisms in an attempt to make sense of the increasingly mad world around me. I'm not unique or unusual, perhaps I'm aware of my limitations, and perhaps I am overly cautious, in the same manner that someone who has been in a nasty car accident would be each time they had to travel. I do keep myself busy in productive ways. I do try to avoid stress at all costs. A stress reaction should come under the category of a nut allergy. I did once want to change the world, rise up and have my voice heard. The world is changing too fast, it doesn't even know what direction it's going in.

I understand that the world owes me nothing, I perhaps understand that better than most. I don't understand why I feel such deep-rooted shame in claiming money from a government who treats us like shit. I feel shame and disgust at where this illness has led me to, the debts, the masquerade, and the constant conflict within me. Eighteen months before I ended up in the psychiatric ward I was doing charity work in Ghana, the Friday before I woke up in the psychiatric ward I had been at a work Christmas party in London. I feel like I was mugged, mugged of a job that paid well, robbed of a house that I loved, friendships became intolerable. I couldn't bear to hear of their normality. Not only was inside my head mad, nothing outside was consistent, safe or familiar.

It has taken nine long years to be able to look life in the eye. I know that I cannot cope with surprise, pressure and stress. I am very cautiously avoiding stress because each time the cracks are repaired you feel weaker, cracks, chips hairline or otherwise leave you weaker, more vulnerable to further damage. While I know that my grasp on reality is currently strong the welfare rights reorganization in the United Kingdom has had a very profound effect on me. I felt a condensed sense of shame. I never knew what it was I wanted to do. I have worked and currently do two voluntary jobs. While I have made a commitment to both of these, I know that both my bosses would understand should I become unwell. I know the corporate world, I understand it, and my brother is a city banker. There would be no compassion from big business or work colleagues especially if an episode lasted a while. A small business wouldn't be able to manage with large numbers of days off. I would feel even more shame and guilt in taking a few days and would never admit to it being anything 'mental health related'. I know from previous experience I would rather make myself ill and not take a day off than fear people thinking or assuming I was 'taking the piss', or god forbid discover the dark secret of my mental illness.

What stability I have is growing from knowing that The Haven is there 24/7. The Haven is different, they help to guide you through the maze of jargon and know when to hold your hand, hold you up when needed and administer a swift metaphorical kick up the arse also. Respect is built, trust earned, based on all aspects of you as a person, not as a curiosity, not as a case study, not an ego trip. It is a delicate balancing act on both sides. It relies on honesty and the ability to take more and more responsibility for your own actions and behaviours, re-learning ways to react to tricky situations, accepting that there is no 'cure', embracing terms like 'management', or 'maintenance' of my condition. Without The Haven I would still be floundering about in the system, lost in the maze of my own thoughts. The stress on my family would continue to be punishing, for both them and me. I would probably have sunk even lower than I thought possible. I have been lost in some dark abysses, but with the support of The Haven there has always been a sense of hope that, within all the despair, I can still get out. There are no tick-boxes that can measure this. It's not just people, and bricks. It's a community built on a mutual ideology, to achieve a 'life worth living' for all involved. We share a sense of pride in who we are, and where we are headed. I know that whatever is thrown at me, with The Haven's help, I can make right choices. They will share in my achievements, and dust me off after a fall. Just knowing that there is a voice of reason at the end of the phone; I think even the most loyal of friends would be sick of me by now. I am slowly winning back the respect of those I hold dear to me. There is no price to be put on that, not for me. Slowly I am being considered an equal, my opinions on various subjects once again considered. My intellectual capacities are no longer being questioned daily.

In other services I have always felt I was never given the time that I needed to reach a constant state of being, always lurching from hyper-manic to depressed. Mainstream psychiatric services would put me together with zombifying medications and construct a house of straw with my life. The Haven has helped me to build solid foundations, and I'm still building. Just like the Little Pigs, I've discovered that a house made of bricks is far more grounded when the wolf of crisis comes knocking.

Moving on: by Rachael Seagrove

It's amazing what a bit love and kindness can do for someone who has grown up it a world that is forever changing; a world which is emotionally and financially demanding; where children could not be children and where the emotional demands were harmful; where adults silenced those around them; where there were footsteps in the middle of the night and shadows on the walls; where it was 'our little secret'. I was the child that was desperate to please and this cost me my innocence. I was that toy that got pulled in every direction, growing up feeling unloved, unheard, learning that the love I had been shown was fake and that the home I grew up in wasn't a home at all. It was four walls, a place where issues were brushed under the carpet, where rules and boundaries didn't exist and Social Services was avoided at all costs.

I soon learnt that my voice didn't count, that a child's words where not believed, were ignored, and that Social Services could allow children to suffer for years leaving them scarred for life and feeling rotten to the core. This made me easy prey for others, made me feel inadequate in front teachers, police officers and my friends, begging for freedom whether that be living or dying, pleading to be put into care for four years. When I was eventually taken into foster care it seems that it was not for my safety, but the safety of my family, because I had become a problem child and account had to be taken of all the stress I had caused the family. My sense of injustice became deep and unforgiving. Again I was punished for something I didn't cause but for something that was done to me and which caused me to lose who I really was. Here were the outer limits of lost identity.

I needed to find a way to FEEL and that came from pulling apart a razor to score my arm with words like evil, bad and the initials of those who harmed me; from the pills in the bottle that I mixed with water and spent my days drinking whilst walking round school with no care for what happened; to sleeping with boys to prove I could; who cares, I don't … I reached 16 years of age and then I was labelled again. I went from being a naughty child, a liar, to 'attention seeking', to being told I had a personality disorder. I was too young to be given this diagnosis. I didn't even know who I was so how could I have a personality that was faulty, that was wrong? I was just me, a child crying out for some love and protection. How was I meant to be, and how was I meant to behave? I didn't know the rules of life. They kept changing from adult to adult, leaving me with no sense of hope. I had given up on myself, but so had everyone else around me, from the doctor who told my parents I would be dead within a year or two, to the teacher who stated that I would never achieve anything.

Whatever I did was wrong, from falling pregnant at 16 to struggling to study in college. The world was against me it felt. I needed saving, but it was my baby daughter who got saved because I couldn't change, I couldn't stop self-harming, I couldn't stop myself from returning to the abuse, I couldn't stop cutting or drinking. Didn't people understand that I was harming myself to survive! My life felt over before it even had a chance to begin and I felt completely out of control, wild and unreachable.

At some point life had to give…to break. I broke…I took a cigarette lighter and put it to my body. I couldn't face the pain anymore. I felt somehow irrevocably flawed and harmful. But I didn't want to harm anyone else, I wanted others to be saved. So I took up that lighter to end my own life but I was not alone in the place where I was staying and I nearly took seven others with me. This was the most soul destroying part that I felt no better than those who had abused and hurt me in the past. I wasn't even 20 and I stood in court pleading guilty to the charge of 'Arson with Intent to Endanger Life'. The only life I had wanted to take away was mine but I had even failed in this. I was left with two options, to live or die, and as dying wasn't working then living it had to be. This wasn't going to be easy and I knew the brick walls would surround me, the rollercoaster feelings would invade me, and low self-esteem would beset me. So how did I build myself back up and who was going to be there without rejecting me?

I needed a purpose. I needed to work. I needed to build my confidence. I was at rock bottom. I had never worked, had never had a job, but I knew I wanted to work. Every job-application I made was rejected. Was it me, my mental health history or the criminal conviction? I felt I was unemployable and for two years I tried and tried to get somewhere, praying someone would give me the chance. I needed a chance to show people what I could do, what I could be and what I could achieve. The Haven had accepted me and cared for me. They had been there and had come to know me when no-one else had. I wanted to give back. I wanted to make a difference. I wanted to use the experiences I had endured, and now understood, to help others to understand. I trained and became a Knowledge and Understanding Framework (KUF) trainer in Personality Disorder (Department of Health 2007). This was my chance for professionals to hear my side of the story, my battle and heartache. This was my chance to make a difference even if it was just to one life, to one person's understanding, to one person's professional practice. I was given the chance and I took it by the horns. Here I was being heard, valued and, most importantly, understood. This was an amazing feeling and I have now helped to train hundreds of mental health and criminal justice professionals in the East of England.

Incredible though this is, somehow it still wasn't enough. I needed to do more. I needed to find a job that accepted me, and my criminal conviction. This felt impossible until I found out about a new service for those with personality disorder that was being created in the next county. I knew deep down in my heart I could do this job. I could be the loving ears for someone who had been hurt like me and I could give that person the chance to just be themselves. I wanted the chance to be an equal. I wanted the chance to share my knowledge, to use my own skills, those I had learned in the most traumatic and authentic way. This job became mine and most of all I got to be part of a team, one where I was respected and listened to. I wasn't judged for the mental illness or criminal conviction. They wanted me and my mistakes. This dream would never have been possible if I hadn't had the chance to come to The Haven who invested time and energy in me, who believed in me and never gave up. They supported me, they listened to me in the darkest of my days, they were there for me when the sun was shining, they became my family they gave me my boundaries, they gave me my voice back and most of all they gave me time. Whether it is day or night, they support me and guide me. I could never put a cost on my life or The Haven because it's so valuable, it's that stunning diamond we all want that sparkles but doesn't dangle with a price tag. You can't put a cost on someone's life, but you can give inspiration and hope.

I am no longer just the girl with a personality disorder. Now I get to learn who I really am because I am not just an illness or a criminal conviction. I am a person. I am also a mother who has miraculously been reunited with her daughter, and I am me.

My perspective as a service user researcher: by Dee Graham

I am not one of the four narrators above. I was the service user selected at The Haven to be the research facilitator for our research focus groups and interviews. I felt an immense sense of privilege was accorded to me by the other service users when they selected me. I had been a researcher prior to the breakdown in my mental health and, re-inspired by Haven research, I have continued to be involved in other research endeavours in the mental health arena, yet The Haven has remained at the heart of what I do. I don't believe it was my research experience that prompted my peers to select me. It is clear from the narratives in this chapter that The Haven is a family and, as an older client, I think that somehow I embodied that maternal, fraternal, or whatever missing family figure might be needed so desperately by others. Our clients at The Haven have not only shared so much with me during research events, they also shared with me when I facilitated our monthly faith group, and while we are out and about on our weekly rambles with the 'pat dog'. All they tell me remains confidential and they know it.

Most of our storytellers in this chapter were involved in Haven core research study and I can identify with all their stories in one way or another: Excluded from help as 'untreatable', lost, alienated and without hope. One of the first tasks I was given at The Haven was to repair the glass in the front door. I saved what stained glass I could and it was in many, many pieces and I realized that there was a certain lack of belief from others that it would ever come together again in one piece. How about that for an analogy of the journey of recovery! But it did come together, with struggle, hard work, and with love, slowly and beautifully. It has a white dove at its centre and, if you would care to take a look again at the image which begins Chapter 3, you will find it pictured there. This was an early step on my journey back to me and in coming to terms with whom and what I am.

I am now in the 'moving on' category, giving talks to students at university, researching, and working with animals at Colchester Zoo. I am so proud to play my part at The Haven and to have witnessed so many remarkable changes for so many people. I am proud to see these journeys committed to print. I think their stories will speak for so many and give hope for the future.

CHAPTER 9

Does the Journey Ever End?

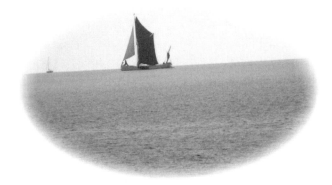

I could never put a cost on my life or The Haven because it's so valuable, it's that stunning diamond we all want that sparkles but doesn't dangle with a price tag.

Service User Quotation

But of course it does have a price tag, one that needs to be sustained on an annual basis. However, before I reveal the more recent events in our story, it is important to review elements of the journey concerning any limitations to our discoveries and it becomes crucial to explore external barriers to progress present in our society. First, following is an examination of comparisons with other recent studies regarding personality and recovery.

When we concluded our study we believed it was the first, internationally, about personality disorder and recovery. However, Katsakou *et al.* (2012) completed a study of recovery in borderline personality disorder which suggested the need for revised treatment targets and outcomes which included priorities important to service users. Also, Zanarini *et al.* (2012) concluded a 16-year study of a large sample of people diagnosed with borderline personality disorder, suggesting that remission of symptoms is more common that full recovery. Both studies concurred with ours in terms of service user involvement in the recovery agenda, and in a concept of recovery not necessarily meaning cure. What is unique about our study is that the significance of the recovery journey in personality disorder has been defined by service users (Castillo, Ramon and Morant 2013). This 20-year journey represents a synergy of different expertise and has been an extraordinary experience of co-production with service users, in both research and service development, one that we hope will inspire others. It is a journey that has also included limitations and barriers.

Risk and trust

The National Evaluation of the 11 community-based personality disorder pilots spoke of the reluctance of some of them to take on people with a forensic history or a dissocial/anti-social personality disorder diagnosis (Crawford 2007). This was not the case at The Haven and, while we judged it important to glean sufficient information about index offences, the vital issue for us was not past offences, but whether the person could be helped to build up trust now and learn to adhere to the boundaries of The Haven as a new service. Table 5.3, Chapter 5 (page 75), shows that 19 of our research participants had a forensic history. This is almost a third of the client sample of the study. Histories ranged from very serious offences to more minor transgressions of the law. During the course of the study a few participants effectively de-registered themselves from the service due to multiple transgressions against The Haven's acceptable behaviour policy. The door was left open, with an opportunity to re-register at the service in the future. Most did re-register.

181

However, two or three clients with a forensic history, who caused untold disturbance at The Haven, are not reflected in research responses because they never became part of the study. In terms of methodological limitations, this was a sampling issue. Ramon *et al.* (2007) stress the importance of personal stories and qualitative approaches to research about recovery, rather than drawing on the 'gold standard' of randomized controlled trials. Therefore, rather than sampling in a randomized way, the need to allow people to choose to participate was most important in this study, which was exploratory in nature. This means that data about the small number of disturbing clients, who we were unable to help, is not directly available from the research. However, it is important to include observations about their differences.

Men are often given a dissocial/anti-social personality disorder diagnosis if they have offended, whilst women tend to retain a borderline categorization (Castillo 2003). Again, whether someone at the service was diagnosed with anti-social/dissocial personality disorder was not the issue because a number who were categorized in this way progressed well. This highlights that it is possible to work well with clients who have been written off by other services or who may have otherwise returned to the criminal justice system. Some clients at the service had a history of violence in other settings, but had never been violent at The Haven and began to make significant progress in their journey of recovery. But the small number of clients under discussion did have a violent forensic history and were diagnosed as dissocial/anti-social. I believe they did not choose to join the research endeavour because their trust was too low to do so. Their sense of betrayal ran so deep that efforts to help them were interpreted as harm and eventually we saw that their fundamental lack of trust gave little chance of them being able to learn the boundaries.

Behaviour for these clients was also influenced by substance misuse; alcohol or opiate use. But, many others at the project had similarly engaged in substance misuse so, again, this was not a factor but rather an exacerbation. Others at the service had displayed damaged aspects of their personality in a dissocial/anti-social way. However, remaining parts of their personality seemed to be more integrated, meaning that a positive side could be appealed to, could learn and could gain dominance over the damaged part. Those we were not able to help appeared to display the damaged aspect of their personality as the dominant side. Although we understood such concepts as transference and projective identification, when someone is threatening to kill you, in realistic terms, or appears determined to destroy the service, it is hard not to take this personally, or not to be disturbed by such behaviour.

It was the service users at The Haven who insisted on de-registration of these clients. In one case, while I was contacting NHS mental health services and the police, clients convened a very large community discussion and insisted I attend until they had reached consensus about de-registration, for they had also been subject to threats and could see clearly how their open community could be damaged by such behaviour. Although this kind of maladaptive behaviour can be understood as a re-enactment of earlier rejection and abuse (Van der Kolk 1989) and what happened could become a further rejection and termination of care, we came to believe that a service must know its limits and protect the greater number of vulnerable people within its walls. We took heart from the words of one carer in our study:

Sammy: Here, for 90 per cent of your clients it's an individual and absolute positive. It ain't going to be for a 100 per cent of people because nothing fits everybody.

When someone, who posed a potential risk to others, was de-registered from The Haven this did not absolve us of responsibility for what happened next. On the rare occasions this happened we requested a professionals meeting. This might result in someone being placed on MAPPA (multi-agency public protection arrangements). It might result in no further action. This begs a question about what happens to the person and the society they are living in. The Henderson Hospital Therapeutic Community for people with a personality disorder diagnosis, in Surrey, England, was as a Tier 4 service, highly specialized for particularly severe and complex cases. It served the south and south east of the country. It was closed down in 2008. If it had been open we would have attempted to refer such clients to this service. There are questions about whether the clients concerned would have been willing to be referred to a Tier 4 service, however, in the consultation which occurred after the closure of the Henderson we responded by saying that we would be likely to refer one person a year to such a service. Many years after its closure, the Henderson is yet to be replaced.

Recent qualitative studies about recovery in forensic settings have been systematically reviewed by Shepherd *et al.* (2015). Their meta-analysis reinforces our findings as they conclude that a key theme, before the recovery process can take place, is a sense of safety and security. They also highlight the fostering of hope and the development of social networks providing a mirror in which personal change can be viewed, thereby establishing personal identity by coming to understand past experience and constructing a sense of self. Although the containing and boundaried experience of a forensic setting is emphasized as a supporting feature, the fear of loss of asylum and the possible toxic nature of some establishments is also identified as a hindrance. The tension inherent in forensic care, in balancing personal autonomy and containment of risk, is also stressed. Shepherd *et al.* call for developments in forensic care that establish a sense of safety and support an understanding of personal identity and, because impending release can pose a threat to both, they advocate the development of social networks during the transition between institutional and community support.

To work or not to work?

In recent decades government policy about mental health in this country has been represented by ten-year plans. New Horizons, the most recent, was created in 2009. Unlike its predecessor, it encompassed the diagnosis of personality disorder and stated that ten times more people in the country had a personality disorder compared to a psychotic disorder such as schizophrenia or bipolar disorder. In this document a former Prime Minister talked of the prejudice and stigma that excludes people with mental health problems from those things that most of us cherish, 'family life, decent homes and careers'. The NHS Performance Framework (Department of Health 2009) came next. This included two new and refreshing outcome indicators for those in mental health care, number in settled accommodation, and number in employment. Hot on the heels of these documents came the Perkins review, *Realizing Ambitions* (Perkins, Farmer and Litchfield 2009), and *Work Recovery and Inclusion* (HMSO 2009), outlining employment support for people in secondary mental health services.

The Perkins review (Perkins *et al.* 2009) was overt in its optimism in a recessionary climate in a country contending with a huge national debt. It claimed that reconfiguration of existing investment could yield more fruitful outcomes. The review highlighted the undesirable consequences of enforced inactivity which robs people of valued roles and networks. It proposed a system of individual placement and support (IPS), a well-researched and successful model of support carried out in the USA and six European countries including England (Bond, Drake and Becker 2008). However, in a study about supported employment for people with mental health problems in the UK (Howard *et al.* 2010) it was found that the effectiveness of IPS was much lower than the success achieved in the US. Results showed that, in those aspiring to employment, there was a 13 per cent success rate, compared to 60 per cent in the US. The study cited differences in the way IPS had been implemented in the UK, and suggested that the disincentives of the UK welfare benefits system, and high unemployment rates in this country, had affected implementation.

McGowan (2009) highlights the fact that the huge complexity of getting people off welfare benefits, and back to work, needs comprehensive solutions and not a one-size-fits-all. For those in secondary care in the NHS, little exists between hospital admissions and the workplace. The lessons of The Haven have shown that a range of leisure and vocational pursuits are needed as building blocks to employment, however, sufficient and appropriate work opportunities need to exist when people are ready for them.

The Perkins review defined employment as ranging from open employment, supported employment, sheltered employment, and sheltered work, to time-limited internships and voluntary work and it looked at the value of work as measured against welfare benefit rates. In addition to support for employees it also addressed employer support in terms of education about mental health 'first-aid'. It talked a great deal about the rights of employees with mental health problems under the Disability Discrimination Act (2005), and the right to reasonable adjustments in working conditions to accommodate mental health difficulties. However, it made only one recommendation about funding for small organizations to cover extended sick leave absences for employees with mental health problems, by using the Access to Work initiative to finance temporary cover for condition-related absences. Similarly, the policy head of the Mental Health Foundation suggested a number of strategies to enable a reversal of a downward trend in employment for people with mental health problems who feel able to begin work (Lawton-Smith 2012). Strategies suggested included the government's Access to Work program. However, BBC News (2014) obtained evidence suggesting that the changes to the government's Access to Work program, with seemingly arbitrary new guidelines introduced then suspended, and widely varying settlements for clients and claims going unpaid for months on end, is denying disabled people the chance to work rather than helping them into employment. Consistent with the Perkins review, Lawton-Smith (2012) also proposed flexible working arrangements, allowing gradual return to work after time off or providing counselling or peer support services, with an emphasis that employers are legally obliged to provide appropriate working arrangements for employees, making 'reasonable adjustments' to prevent disabled employees from being disadvantaged at work. I would like to suggest that some employers may be afraid to employ those with a mental health history because they fear being sued under the Disability Discrimination

Act. Even if an organization is too small to be expected to make reasonable adjustments a case can still be brought under the Disability Discrimination Act, and there is a cost, in terms of both legal fees and stress, in fighting this at an Employment Tribunal. Even when an employer is a caring one, financial viability remains a crucial and necessary concern that is likely to remain hidden because any concern is currently seen as discriminatory. In point of fact, research has suggested that less than 40 per cent of employers would consider employing someone with a mental health problem (Lawton-Smith 2012).

In Chapter 8 our four service user narrators had differing aspirations in their journey of recovery; our first narrator pursued freedom, voluntary work and travel; for the second it was inclusion in countryside activities and the family; for the fourth narrator it was paid employment and all that meant in terms of teamwork and self-value. She had been deprived of a career because of the circumstances of her life and, against all the odds, obtained employment for the first time. However, the journey of our third narrator highlights social contexts, in terms of the current economic climate and opportunities, which continue to impact on her journey. Our third narrator, who had at one time been in employment, voiced a perspective echoed by older participants in our research who had previously been in employment:

Helen: I am very cautiously avoiding stress because each time the cracks are repaired you feel weaker, cracks, chips hairline or otherwise leave you weaker, more vulnerable to further damage.

Beresford (2013) believes that globalization and the drive to free market economies is creating oppression for people with mental health problems which is expanding into many countries. This includes the countries of the UK where 'reforms' are creating a welfare system that is becoming painful to negotiate, where capacity tests are increasing in frequency and where public services are being reduced.

Helen: The welfare rights reorganization in the United Kingdom has had a very profound effect on me...I don't understand why I feel such deep-rooted shame in claiming money from a government who treats us like shit.

While some may say that we must insist on reasonable employment adjustments and challenge stigma, our third narrator makes astute observations about the lack of compassion from big business and the lack of financial ability of small businesses to accommodate such adjustments.

Helen: I have worked, and currently do two voluntary jobs. While I have made a commitment to both of these, I know that both my bosses would understand should I become unwell. I know the corporate world...there would be no compassion from big business or work colleagues especially if an episode lasted a while. A small business wouldn't be able to manage with large numbers of days off.

Safeguards need to work both for the employee *and the employer*, and they need to be clearly enshrined within the law. If not, I predict that a sufficient number of employers will not become available to employ those with mental health problems. If a reconfiguration of existing investment can yield more fruitful outcomes (Perkins *et al.* 2009) this is not yet occurring in any meaningful way. This would require sufficient investment in a wide range of occupational activities, including supported work, sheltered placements and social firms, for those with mental health difficulties, and a true understanding that some people with mental health problems need to work in a less stressful way.

187

What happened next at The Haven?

The Bradley Report (Department of Health and Ministry of Justice 2009) was Lord Bradley's independent review of people with mental health problems in the criminal justice system. The many recommendations of the report included early intervention coupled with community support and prevention. This was a response to the growing consensus that prison may not always be the best environment for people with personality disorder because it can exacerbate mental health problems, self-harm and suicidality. The review highlighted that the majority of offenders with mental health disorders are not dangerous and could be better treated outside the prison system without any risk to the public. The Department of Health, in conjunction with the Ministry of Justice National Offender Management Service, engaged in a consultation exercise regarding what should be done in response to the Bradley Report. By October 2011 they had published their *Response to the Offender Personality Disorder Consultation* which represented a new national strategy for the management of mentally disordered offenders.

In November 2011, just a few short weeks before Christmas, I was called to a meeting at the Department of Health in London, together with the other national personality disorder project leads. Here we were told that a new national strategy for offenders had just been signed off by ministers. Although this could not be interpreted as anything but good news for the growing numbers of people with a personality disorder diagnosis who had become trapped in the criminal justice system, it was news which came to us with disquieting implications. For we were told that this meant that funding which had, up until now, been used for the national personality disorder projects, would begin to be diverted into the criminal justice system to finance the new offender strategy. The news was received at the meeting by those around the table quite soberly I thought. Apart from me that is … 'Hang on a minute…hang on a minute'. My primary thought was that The Haven, as the only national project entirely in the voluntary sector, was very vulnerable indeed. Only two years before, as outlined in Chapter 7, local commissioners had refused to provide the £60,000 per annum needed for The Haven social inclusion unit. In light of this new development, how would they respond to a request for £600,000? This would be ten times as much, sought at a time when the government was introducing austerity measures and launching a spending review, synonymous with 'funding will be as scarce as hen's teeth'. After the meeting I was seen separately and assured that the last thing The Department of Health wanted to see was the closure of The Haven and I was promised consultancy help to guide us through negotiations with local commissioners aimed to preserve our future.

I returned to Colchester and told no-one. The news was a ringing silence within me. This was an announcement that could be a bit of a Christmas-spoiler and it felt best not to disclose it until after the festive season. Haven Christmas parties were wondrous affairs. The staff would choose a secret theme for fancy dress for the team. Clients would come dressed as they liked. Some of them came, transformed, in ball gowns and suits and bowties. The food was always a splendid spread, but mostly these parties were full of love and so much fun. It was not unusual for clients to say it was the best Christmas they ever had. To me, they were just the best. That year we had a Cinderella theme. Although the ugly sisters were stunning, and there was even a third dressed in drag, it is the pumpkin that sticks in my mind as the most hilarious. The staff member in question interviewed a new and rather serious client, in full pumpkin garb, complete with bright orange face. This was also the year that, during the party, Cinders got called to the police station to support one of our clients who had been arrested. She told the police officers, 'The choice was me, a pumpkin or an ugly sister.' I was dressed as the Fairy Godmother, dispensing cheer, although my heart took pause as I remembered our new situation. It was like someone was trying to write The Haven's story in a different way, a way not intended. As the partygoers danced and joyfully sang, 'I would go five hundred miles,' to onlookers I blithely gave out raffle prizes but felt, in truth, that I would need to be a fairy godmother, for real, to get us out of this one.

As the New Year approached I began to feel more optimistic and more prepared for the disclosure of our situation to the Board of Directors. After all, our track record was exemplary. After all, we had comprehensive research evidence of our effectiveness. After all, we had service and cost savings evidence. And after all, The Bradley Report spoke of the development of an inter-departmental strategy for the management of all levels of personality disorder within both the health service and the criminal justice system. Surely we would become a part of this. Surely it would not be wise to develop a new framework which dismantled existing and effective prevention structures in the process. However, all national personality disorder project leads then received a letter stating in stark terms that our central funding would now begin to taper off…we were to be decommissioned. I informed the Chairman of The Haven Board and he set up a new sub-committee for funding comprising some of The Haven Directors. The news still remained concealed and the staff team would not be made aware of it until June 2012. The service users were not told until October that year. After many years of collaboration with service users we stepped into the future without our long-established modus operandi of co-production.

Monthly funding meetings began. By spring, true to their word, the Department of Health sent a consultant to join the funding committee to support us in the process. By summer, the Department of Health assured us that central funding would be made available for The Haven until 2015. This was an opportunity to inform Haven managers and the staff team, giving the assurance that we had over two years to solve the problem. The funding committee spoke of raising money from organizations like

189

the Big Lottery. I had always been keen to source additional funding from charitable organizations for the social inclusion unit and other new initiatives, however, finding over half a million pounds sterling each year, to sustain core services, is a daunting prospect and I felt that we were providing a valuable health service which should be paid for by the health economy. Nevertheless, I attended workshops hosted by the local volunteer bureau, aimed at learning how to put together bids and tenders. I sat together with voluntary sector personnel, physical disability, brain-injury and others. Good people all fretting about their organizations and their clients. At one workshop I said to the man from the county council that there would be no voluntary sector left in the district if matters proceeded in this way. Someone had to say it. At this point his cheerful façade fractured as he lamented the funding cuts the local authority was being subjected to. Tangible fear spread around the room.

I began to meet and get to know the people who would be manning the new health commissioning structures. PCTs (Primary Care Trusts) were due to be replaced by CCGs (Clinical Commissioning Groups) by April 2013. One friendly CCG member said to me, 'You know the trouble is, Heather, that you don't belong to anyone.' My thought was that we did indeed belong to someone, we belonged to our clients. However, there it was again, a reminder of our voluntary sector vulnerability. Meantime, the funding committee at The Haven decided that we needed a business manager. We had insufficient allocation in our staffing budget to employ a business manager, but the committee felt it would be better to overspend on this to secure our future funding. The new business manager joined the funding committee and, together with him, I attended our first meeting with the forming CCG. At the meeting we were given advice and pointers on how to pitch our business case to the new commissioners.

As a learning organization (Senge 1990), engaged in co-production with its service users, up until now our collective aspirations had been set free and we had learned to see the whole together, adapting to our circumstances as the organization grew and developed. However, it was now only the professionals at The Haven who knew of our uncertain future and the potential precipice that lay before us two years hence. Capacity was an issue we had always adapted to and, as our client numbers grew, the need for more crisis/respite beds now became very evident. Uncharacteristically without consultation with Haven clients, I had a wall built across an upstairs room with two windows and created a fifth bedroom. My instincts were to carry out a loft-conversion, which would give us three more bedrooms, and to rent external premises for the growing social inclusion initiative, thereby demarcating more clearly the progress between those in need of a great deal of crisis and therapeutic support, and those now more externally focused on life outside of The Haven. For anyone reading this who is engaged in service development, it is important to note that such an organization as The Haven, with a relatively small staff team, could support more crisis/respite beds than four. I believe that seven or eight would be possible in such a structure. The staff team consisted of two part-time social inclusion staff, two full-time day staff, and a part-time administrator and a finance officer. Additionally, eight staff, two for each out-of-hours shift, manned the 24/7 part of the service, backed up by a team of bank workers for occasional shifts that might need to be filled. It was from this time that I noted the staff team becoming stressed and tired, particularly the day staff. This could have been construed as a capacity problem, however, I believe this change in morale was due to the shifting ground beneath our feet which made it more difficult to build on earlier successes. Where previously we had been a machine focused on risk and personal development, and all the stages in-between, the funding situation was now a constant distraction.

In October 2012 all Haven clients were invited to an open meeting called, 'Where there's tea there's hope'. The meeting concerned The Haven and its future funding. A central and distressing issue for me at this time was the fear that I had helped to lead a group of such vulnerable people, desperately in need of love and stability, to a point where they truly believed in our transitional recovery ethos. They trusted that their newly developed healthy attachment would not be taken away. What idealism I had helped to foster in such an uncertain world. Encompassed within my personal idealism was the belief that, if something was so workable and so successful, no-one could possibly take it away. Despite all my fears about the reaction of our service users, the community of Haven clients responded well to the news and resolved to *find a way to show those who hold the purse strings how The Haven is helping each and every one of us*. After this meeting, at last, the client lead was invited onto the funding committee which now proceeded in the more comfortable mode of shared decision-making.

The consensus at the funding committee was that we needed to ask local funders for more money, not less, because less than one asked for was usually what was forthcoming. Also, because we were growing in

191

client numbers, the funding committee wanted us to move to much larger premises. I began to feel out-of-step with the committee. It seemed to me that, in such a climate, we needed to consolidate what we had and I could see how we could make our current space work. Some of the committee characterized this as me being too attached to our premises in Glen Avenue. Certainly I cared about the place, but to our clients it was the brick mother (Rey 1994). It was a crucial aspect of the first levels of our pyramid of progress and one not easy to replace in such uncertain times. However, it was imagination and dreams that had begun this journey and now it felt that it would soon be time for those younger than me to carry forward those dreams.

The business manager was tasked with creating a business plan which would take our remaining two years funding and spread it over four years, tapering each year, with a request to the Clinical Commissioning Group (CCG) to pick up the annual shortfall until The Haven became transferred to local funding. Meantime, the usual activities continued at The Haven. In 2010 we had begun to co-ordinate the KUF initiative for the East of England. The KUF is the personality disorder knowledge and understanding training framework, that is, a training initiative created by a group of very experienced and accomplished professionals and service users, and funded by the Department of Health (2007). Uniquely, awareness level courses required that one trainer should be a professional and the other a service user with a personality disorder diagnosis. This was a tremendously successful initiative for us and, by 2013, with the support of statutory and voluntary training partners in Essex, Suffolk, Norfolk and Bedfordshire, over 750 professionals in the Eastern Region of England had graduated from personality disorder KUF awareness level courses. The implications of the Bradley Report (Department of Health and Ministry of Justice 2009) also meant that this initiative would eventually be affected because KUF funds for the training of mental health staff were to be diverted to criminal justice staff. Anticipating this, we began to run courses for probation teams and prison staff with equal success.

Additionally, The Haven had a tradition of sharing lessons about the service. Each month we ran an Open Day afternoon and visitors came from near and far. By this time other aspiring personality disorder services were beginning to be developed, using aspects of The Haven service. This included areas like Liverpool, and the Waves Project set up in the next county by Suffolk Mind, also the Lighthouse Project in Brighton created by the Sussex Mental Health Trust. Ensuring service user ownership, their clients were at the heart of decision-making and service provision. Other countries also called on our lessons and our policies in their aspirations to build personality disorder services, including a personality disorder champion for Western Australia who said that the pinnacle of her visit to the UK was discovering The Haven. On behalf of The Haven, I became involved in a collaboration to put together a new National Personality Disorder Practitioner Guide (Department of Health 2014) and it was rewarding to see inclusions, from both of our research studies, among the service user quotations contained in the guide. Although the future might be uncertain, we continued to do what we had always done. We stepped onward constructively.

On behalf of the funding committee, the business manager submitted a very sound business plan to the CCG in January 2013, which included clear evidence for future cost-savings to the health economy. In May 2013 the CCG called us around the table, together with the local Mental Health Trust, with the purpose of looking at The Haven's business plan. I was surprised to see former PCT staff at the meeting, who had in the past not shown much interest or support for The Haven, now acting as advisors to the new CCG. At the meeting the Mental Health Trust was very complementary and respectful of Haven services. However, the CCG stated that there was no remaining funding for Haven core costs. Our service user lead was present at the meeting and I believe she then truly began to comprehend the seriousness of our situation, creating a burden she would shoulder for the foreseeable future. Although not explicitly said at the meeting, my belief was that the CCG wished the Mental Health Trust to consider absorbing The Haven and its funding. Despite the Mental Health Trust's appreciation of our service, I felt there was little chance of this occurring because they, like other NHS Mental Health Trusts in the country, had been tasked with saving £40 million. I believed that they had cut back significantly over the past five years in relation to staff, hospital beds and resources and they felt this had not been acknowledged. Although we might save the Mental Health Trust money in the future, they were caught in the NHS conundrum of spending less money now only to pay more in the long run. Finally, the CCG advised they would not be willing to spend public money without a full investigation and verification of cost savings and the development of a clear personality disorder pathway.

Independent consultants were commissioned by the CCG to investigate and compile a report about the pathway. Both the Mental Health Trust and The Haven were interviewed and tasked with providing comprehensive data. Haven clients threw themselves into this process wholeheartedly and invited the consultant, carrying out the review, to a meeting at The Haven where they spoke from the heart about all their service meant to them and what it had done for them. I compiled a 29-page pathway document with attendant files. We poured everything we knew about our service into the process. Once this was finished, a few days before my 65th birthday, I retired as Haven Chief Executive on 15 November 2013. By December the independent consultant report had been completed and was made available (Abley 2014). The Haven business manager kindly forwarded me a copy. It represented Haven services in glowing terms and made reference to the key outcome of The Haven's remarkable suicide record, despite suicide rates for this client group being very high. Excerpts from the report read as follows:

> North East Essex currently appears to have an above average level of service provision for people with personality disorder. In fact it could be argued that the service received by some clients through a combination of The Haven and North Essex Mental Health Partnership Trust is exceptional in comparison to those receiving generic local mental services for other mental health problems. The leadership of The Haven is to be commended and their unrelenting commitment to the development and delivery of such exceptional local services for those with personality disorder. As these local services now stand they offer a substantial potential legacy to the local health economy. (Abley 2014, p.24)

One point in the report that puzzled me was the lack of information regarding the cost of out-of-area placements. Each year a number of patients with mental health problems prove to be so problematic and risky that they are placed in secure and specialist hospitals out of the area, usually private sector hospitals, and usually at great cost to the local NHS. Such patients have often attracted a personality disorder diagnosis. It seemed to me that, because of the existence of The Haven, a comparison of the cost of out-of-area placements for North East Essex would measure most favourably against the other NHS areas in Mid Essex and West Essex. However, the consultant report simply stated that this information was not available.

In response to enquiries regarding The Haven's future, the client lead received a letter from the CCG in February 2014. In it the CCG said, that while recognizing the importance of the service provided by The Haven, they wanted to be assured that they commissioned services that provided high quality care, delivered the best possible outcomes and also provided excellent value for money, using a collaborative approach working with existing providers to create a dedicated care pathway. However, the independent consultant report stated the following in relation to the existing pathway:

> *The Haven already forms an integral part of the North East Essex personality disorder treatment pathway. If The Haven were no longer in existence, a significant number of personality disordered clients would require support, crisis interventions and an ongoing and potentially intensive containment function which would have to be provided through existing resources at North Essex Mental Health Partnership Trust. (Abley 2014, p.23)*

In the letter of 24 February 2014, to The Haven client lead, the CCG also stated their intention to run a procurement exercise in 2014 with the expectation that a five-year contract would be awarded to the successful bidder in January 2015.

A political backdrop to developments

When I began my career in mental health at the beginning of the 1990s, the management and funding structures of the health sector were relatively simple ones. Born of Aneurin Bevan's National Health Service established in 1948, uncomplicated frameworks had endured. The Secretary of State for Health was in charge of the Department of Health and structures were straightforward, with Regions and District Health Authorities. For those of us on the front lines of service delivery the channels of accountability were clear. At that time, in North East Essex, the voluntary sector was strong with a relatively large number of mental health organizations working alongside the NHS. I don't wish to sugar-coat the quality of mental health services back then, for we had much to learn about patient rights and workable services, however, the system was tightly integrated and our funders were accessible. It was quite usual for the local mental health commissioner to bring the mental health voluntary sector together into one room and listen to our needs and wants. At such meetings people would make known, for example, that more help was needed for alcohol services or that advocacy services needed to be better funded. Public consultation is now the current ethos and I have attended public meetings in recent years

195

where opportunities were given for views to be expressed. However, in earlier years, it was a much more intimate experience where funders had a hands-on knowledge of the services in their area and where, albeit a little paternalistically, we were listened to and responded to with action. There was nothing tokenistic about it.

In was during the 1990s that a Conservative government began to advocate a primary-care-led NHS with Primary Care General Practitioner (GP) capacity to purchase secondary health care services. Commissioning functions were split by creating 'purchasers' and 'providers' in the local health system (National Health and Community Care Act 1990). This began to create two models of commissioning, one based on health authorities, and the other based on general practice with fund-holding GPs who had the ability to purchase non-urgent community care for their patients. In 1999 Alan Milburn became Secretary of State for Health in a New Labour government which introduced legislation (National Health Service Reform and Health Care Professions Act 2002) that was to dissolve old commissioning structures and place power more fully into the arena of general practice by creating Primary Care Trusts (PCTs). PCTs were free standing bodies, accountable to Regional Health Authorities, holding 80 per cent of the health budget. Now the door to privatization, opened by the previous government, was pushed a little wider. To its credit, under New Labour, the NHS did make some significant progress during the early part of the millennium, including reductions in hospital waiting times and a drop in infant mortality. In the mental health field there was an increase in access to specialist services and the introduction of crisis intervention and resolution teams, some considered to be among the best in Europe, leading to reductions in acute psychiatric hospital admissions (Thorlby and Maybin 2010). This was a time when innovation was encouraged and although Alan Milburn left his position as Secretary of State for Health in 2003, which was the year before The Haven was to open, we were I believe a service born of that era.

Despite the prevailing 'change-culture' of successive governments, in the early days of The Haven our commissioning relationships were good. Little had changed for us as we were being centrally funded and we maintained a fruitful alliance with the National Personality Disorder Team at the Department of Health. Our funding channelled via the newly formed PCT structures. However, because Mental Health Services were considered to be a fairly specialist function, the commissioning for the whole of North Essex was given to a lead-commissioning PCT, West Essex. This was staffed by former Health Authority personnel who we knew well. Although there would be requests for items like carbon footprint plans and infection control policies, where with a sign and a moan about bureaucracy we would break off from the business of preventing suicides to put them in place, basically they were sound requests. Service level agreements (service contracts) were forthcoming, meetings and visits were frequent and we felt that the PCT really cared about our service. After a few years the lead commissioning function transferred to another PCT in the area. No service level agreements were forthcoming and visits never occurred, not once. The PCT became a funding conduit only. Whether this was a lack of interest coupled with the increasing complexity of commissioning structures, leaving the lead commissioning PCT little time for familiarization with services being commissioned, I am not really sure. It was during these latter years that I saw the erosion of the mental health voluntary sector in our area with many services disappearing. We counted ourselves very fortunate to be centrally funded by the National Personality Disorder Team at the Department of Health.

William Beverage designed the NHS during the Second World War. Its underpinning principle was to raise money according to income and redistribute it according to need, ensuring health care for all. Even at that time politicians said it could not be afforded. Beverage (1942) said, however, that the failure to abolish want before the war was a 'needless scandal' and one which was easily within the country's economic resources to prevent. The British NHS went on to become a model for the rest of the world for more than 50 years. From 1948 onwards, health care costs in this country remained around three to four per cent of the GDP, that is, the gross domestic product, or output, of the country, divided by its population. Appleby (2013) attributes the growing cost of health care in the country to a growing population, growth in national wealth, increases in the costs of providing care, and developments in medical technology. Predicting a future increase in health care, which will be of benefit to the nation and its productivity, he puts forward the consideration of possible trade-offs with other government spending. However, Pollock (2014) suggests that significant increases in the percentage of GDP spent on health care costs did not start to occur until the 1990s, when privatization in the NHS began to take place. Privatization occurred under successive governments and even well after his tenure as Secretary of State for Health,

Alan Milburn continued to be a proponent of competition in the NHS and an advocate for the entrance of wider commercial partners (Ramesh 2011).

The Health and Social Care Act (2012) was then launched by the coalition government of Conservatives and Liberal Democrats. Pollock (2014) characterizes this as the 'destructive bill' or the 'abolishing act'. She compares the slim document, which was the 1946 NHS Act, with the 457 pages of legal and technical detail which constitute the current Health and Social Care Act. In two of those pages, what the new act does is to remove the 60-year duty of the Secretary of State to provide health care for all. The act introduces insurance structures based on US lines and gives powers to create a market of private providers who can pick and choose which patients will receive care and what they will charge for it. When the Act was introduced I was foolish enough to think this might open the door to more services being provided by the voluntary sector or what is now often known as the 'third sector' (a term which prophetically suggested that it would be third in the pecking-order). However, rather than voluntary sector opportunities, what we are seeing is the introduction of big business, corporate providers. There has been a plethora of postings on social media regarding donations received by MPs who voted in parliament for privatization of the NHS, donations from the corporate health world. This caused one person to post a suggestion that, like racing drivers, MPs should wear clothes which advertise the logos of their 'sponsors'.

Additionally, within the complexity of the social care debate I have heard arguments about what is health care, what is social care and about the integration of health and social care. To me it is a tennis match where no-one wants the funding ball to fall in their court. Pollock (2014) points out that the vertical delegation of power in the NHS, within simple and integrated systems, has now been replaced by the bureaucracy of the market, a plethora of new bodies, including CCGs which she characterizes as nothing more than insurance funds created on US lines. She warns of an NHS which will be hollowed out to remain as a logo only and a future of excess administration costs, unnecessary commercially marketed treatments, missed prevention opportunities and the exclusion of complex needs.

During much of the time since The Haven's business plan was submitted to the new CCG, our local General Hospital has been in and out of 'special measures', that is, failure to meet acceptable measures of health care because of substandard performance, especially concerning cancer patients. This matter has frequently been on regional television news and also the national news with the Secretary of State for Health standing outside the Houses of Parliament at Westminster, talking about difficulties at Colchester General Hospital. It is not hard to guess, in such circumstances, where our local CCGs attention has been drawn. But, is our local general hospital inefficient or simply starved of funds, meaning insufficient staff members who are free enough from administration tasks, and target-attainment, to carry out the function of healing?

Ramon (2011) highlights a multiplicity of cycles of imposed change in NHS organizations. This is exacerbated by the politics of self-interest. It was Nye Bevan who said, at the inception of the NHS in 1948, that it will last as long as there are folk left with the faith to fight for it. In November 2014, thousands of people in this country petitioned, and wrote to their MPs, in support of the National Health Service (Amended Duties and Powers) Bill, which was read in parliament with the intention of beginning to roll back privatization in the NHS. The bill was passed. On the day there was little coverage by the media, which concerned itself rather with the current details of party politics in light of impending elections. However, the next day the petitioners secured a whole page of The Guardian newspaper saying 'We heart the NHS' and highlighted the issues. Lucas (2014) stresses the fact that, although this is a step in the right direction, the bill does not go far enough. She suggests that it will take vision and swift, collective action to rescue the NHS from the privateers. A second private members' bill has now been proposed, the NHS Reinstatement Bill (Roderick and Pollock 2014). This bill, if it ever reaches parliament, provides a template for necessary reinstatement and reform and addresses the failures of the 2012 Health and Social Care Act. It would reinstate the government's legal duty to provide the NHS in this country; re-establish district health authorities; and abolish competition and marketization, allowing commercial companies to provide services only if the NHS and its networks could not do so, resulting in suffering for patients. It would also prohibit ratification of the Transatlantic Trade and Investment Partnership (TTIP), preventing free trade agreements between governments of two or more countries resulting in transnational corporations gaining the right to enter the UK health market and operate without limits on their activities.

Where does The Haven sit in this political realm? It is a microcosm of need and its lobbying for survival becomes lost in the global picture. But a microcosm is crucially indicative of how the vulnerable are responded to in our corporate world. Monbiot (2014) suggests that global corporate power is the key political issue of our age which limits the scope of democracy. It is distorting spending, it explains the creeping privatization of health and it has left public services with unpayable debts.

The wheel has come full circle

It is precious to me that I have been part of such a community as The Haven. Part of healing is to come together in community and one of the best things about a community is that it enables us to work together, sharing strengths and responsibilities while valuing each other. In The Good Ship Haven many people shared the helm. My ten years with The Haven were probably the most rewarding, and the most exhausting, of my life. Never have I had a team who worked so hard or service users who were so committed and involved in an endeavour. In particular, the latter years of balancing the priorities of saving and enhancing lives with the search to secure future funding, were punishing. After retiring as chief executive I had the time to gain some perspective about the climate I had worked in during those last two years. I could see that, in my heart, I had known we were playing against an increasingly stacked deck. My successor assumed the role of chief executive. I wanted to maintain my link with The Haven and its clients, my contact with the community, so I continued as a weekly sessional therapist running the life skills group. In February 2014, in an effort to demonstrate to commissioners a willingness to cut back and to pare down the service to perceived basic necessities, the sessional therapists at The Haven were discontinued and, much to my regret, me along with them.

I began to volunteer a day each week at the social inclusion unit's outdoor well-being program and what a joy that has been. Together with Haven clients who have joined us down on the farm, we have gardened, cut and worked with willow, rambled through wild flower meadows, pressed apples and many other activities. As I have looked up at the oak trees on the horizon, seen the birds flying over the water, and watched the crops turn from green to gold, I have thought that, if this makes me feel so good, it reinforces all my beliefs about what a very healing experience this can be for service users, helping mood, morale and confidence so much. Whatever happens to The Haven this is a part of the service that could be sustained, working in collaboration with other green-care partners. I tell the clients down on the farm about a service in an adjacent town which began in the

1990s when advocates and service users set up a series of self-help groups at the advocacy offices, for all diagnoses not just personality disorder. When I left to work in the advocacy service in Colchester the self-help groups decided to take their £10,000 funding and become independent from Mind, adopting the title of the Mayday Self-Help Groups. Running on a shoe-string budget, and operated with peer support, over 20 years later they have survived. So I tell the clients at the farm that I believe, when people care about each other enough, and are determined enough, it is possible to survive. My hope is that the outdoor well-being program will survive together with additional aspects of The Haven and its social inclusion unit, a little phoenix egg, together with the lessons of The Haven and its research, ready to hatch and grow during better times.

Adlam *et al.* (2012) have opened a discourse regarding the internal pitfalls and challenges to services who work with severe personality disorder. They also reflect on the demise of some established organizations such as The Henderson Hospital, suggesting this was due to an oversimplification of the notion of the psychological complexities of personality disorder on the part of commissioners (Wrench 2012). These are words that I believe will come home to roost, nationally and regionally. An exemplar: In 2014, the chief clinical officer of North East Essex CCG claimed that The Haven did not reach sufficient local residents in the area suffering from personality disorder (Porter 2014). Yes, this is correct. The Haven did not reach all in the area with personality disorder which would amount to well in excess of 16,000 people. It did, however, reach the most severe and risky among them. The CCG claims to be working on a long-term strategy to ensure the needs of local people with personality disorder are met. This would require massive investment, far in excess of Haven funding. I predict that this will be as 'successful' a commissioning pledge as many others, with short-termism at its heart.

It remains true that the world is still full of want and war, that health services are only one part of an endangered welfare situation, that mental health services are one part of health services, and that personality disorder is one aspect of mental health services. However, people with a personality disorder diagnosis have been highlighted as a client group that suffers significant social exclusion which has a high impact on health and other public services (Social Exclusion Task Force 2006) and what the National Personality Disorder Program achieved for those with this diagnosis, during the ten years it was funded, was significant and genuinely avant-garde. Today, of the 11 community pilots, one was for adolescents, remaining centrally funded; some have now closed after central funding came to an end; others situated within Mental Health Trusts have fared variously, some have been pared down and are less than their former selves; and a minority have flourished in a well-established and diversified way.

In recent months, while engaged in talks and service development sessions in other areas, I have been asked to explain what The Haven has done wrong to find itself in the current funding predicament when it has been looked at by so many areas as a model for the future for personality disorder services. I tell them, nothing that I know of. I am also asked what will happen if it closes and whether, as usual, NHS mental health services will be expected to mop up the fall-out. The local Mental Health Trust recently held a meeting with Haven clients to assure them that, if the service closes, they will provide support and a help-line for any who are still registered with the Mental Health Trust. While commendable, this will of course encourage a number of service users to take steps in the direction of statutory services when they had been walking in another direction for some years. I spoke to two nurses from the local psychiatric inpatient unit recently. They told me that now the wards are increasingly admitting Haven clients.

At the end of 2014, The Haven client lead said to me that she felt The Haven was in a coma and she was sitting by its bedside wondering if it was going to die, or make a full or partial recovery. No procurement exercise by the local CCG, to award the promised contract in January 2015, has materialized. The new chief executive has tried hard, against many obstacles and Haven clients have instigated a media campaign with coverage on local TV news and newspapers, local and national. In one national newspaper, The Haven client lead expressed astonishment at the Deputy Prime Minister's call for a Zero Suicides Action Plan when he is part of a coalition government which has introduced the very cuts that have affected The Haven, *'I want to tell him, look at the projects that work. We're doing what we are meant to be doing and what works, but you are closing us. They say we're mad and yet this is corporate insanity'* (Wynne-Jones 2015). Campaigning, lobbying and fundraising efforts are taking place, hoping for a case of brinkmanship with a reprieve at the 11th hour. Currently, it is a bleak prospect to look at the fundraising page edging to its first few thousands when it is hundreds of thousands of pounds which are being sought.

We thought our journey was about hopes and dreams and working together to find new ways, treatments and services. But in the end it was about politics and commissioning. And is there an ending to this story, or is this simply the place where I have stopped writing it?

Have you thought of an ending?

Yes, several, and all are dark and unpleasant.

Oh, that won't do! Books ought to have good endings. How would this do: and they all settled down and lived together happily ever after?

It will do well, if it ever came to that.

Ah! And where will they live? That's what I often wonder.

Tolkien (1954, p.226)

In February, 2015, The Haven at Glen Avenue had to close its doors to its clients.

Appendices

Appendix I Research Timeline

Date	Method	Duration of data analysis	Duration of formal data collection	Duration of SEGs	Duration of other background data/minutes	Duration of numerical data collection	Duration of research group
June 04	Creation of the research group						
July 04	Collection of numerical data						
July 04	Other background data						
Feb 05	Service evaluation group (SEG)						
May 05	Service evaluation group (SEG)						
Aug 05	Service evaluation group (SEG)						
Nov 05	Service evaluation group (SEG)						
Feb 06	Service evaluation group (SEG)						
May 06	Service evaluation group (SEG)						

Aug 06	First client focus group				
Aug 06	First of 20 client interviews				
Nov 06	Second client focus group				
Feb 07	Third client focus group				
Mar 07	First carer focus group				
May 07	Fourth client focus group				
July 07	Last of 20 client interviews				
Aug 07	Second carer focus group				
Aug 07	Service evaluation group (SEG)				
Nov 07	Service evaluation group (SEG)				
Nov 07	Data analysis begins				
June 09	Data analysis ends				
Sept 09	Last meeting of the research group				

Appendix II Research Group
Diary 2004–2009

Friday 25 June 2004

At the very first research group there were nine people present and we began with an introduction to the aims of The Haven. We have started at temporary premises at the Northgate Centre and we're looking for a permanent home. Meantime we're only open during the day. Heather explained that the aim of the research is to look at how and why The Haven Project is effective over the two years of the pilot. It will be follow-on from previous local research. There will be training for service user researchers and payment will be made within the confines of the therapeutic earnings limits as set by the Department of Work and Pensions; this will ensure that user researchers' welfare benefit entitlements are not compromised, whilst ensuring fair recompense for work carried out.

The group talked about a couple of papers that had been written concerning recovery within mental health and discussed the concept of recovery, with recovery being a journey, not an imposed pressure to get well. Most members of the group agreed that recovery is not the word that they would choose to use. Those who are moving out of mental illness, particularly those with a PD diagnosis do not want to recover who they were, they want to get to a future that they want and what they think everyone else has. They want to disregard all the pain and problems of the past and all that happened to them and to become new, maybe to be reborn, not to go back to all that was wrong in the first place. We discussed the term iatrogenic, that is, harm caused by something that is supposed to do good, in this case the health care services and it was agreed that psychiatric services can be iatrogenic. We looked at methods to recover and some of the ideas brought up were: hope, independence and empowerment (medical treatments, e.g. drugs can impede recovery).

People at the group felt the need to feel safe and discussed the question: What makes us feel safe? Quality of life is important, as is restoring the ability to cope with life; positive coping strategies would be very useful. Independence is a goal, but remembering that interdependence is also important, we all need to depend on others. It is part of the human condition, and so it is unreasonable to expect someone to be totally independent and, as such, it is an unrealistic goal. The idea of adult babysitting for people in crisis or those feeling particularly vulnerable was discussed. It was felt that therapeutic alliances are very important, as are consistent respectful relationships with staff. A national anti-stigma campaign is needed.

We then looked at what sort of questions could be asked by researchers to determine whether The Haven Project has been successful, staying with the idea of recovery, the following points were raised:

- It's not getting back to the way you were.
- It's about growing and overcoming challenges.
- Hope, independence, empowerment.

How does it feel for you?

- expectations
- what didn't work before?
- optimisms – where in 5 years?
- what has worked?
- inner progress?
- scales – sliding
- inner calm and anxieties
- safety net
- coping strategies
- what have you learnt?
- changed behaviour and reasons for behaviour
- do you like yourself?
- occupation
- strengths – looking for positives and futures
- qualities.

Finally we looked at what support needs to be in place for people using The Haven Project, these are the ideas we had, although we welcome any new ones:

- sweetie chute – candy
- encouragement
- staff that are different – non-judgemental
- part of community
- a quiet place – set it aside

- comfort – calm décor

- homely

- normal

- common ground

- problem-free room

- golden phone call

- bright room

- activities – different to others already offered

- support groups for those ready for them.

Friday 31 July 2004

Four people attended the meeting. Some measures regarding outcomes were discussed including the Ohio study, as recommended by Piers Allott 'NIMHE Recovery Fellow', this details a different concept of recovery.

Eight people have registered with The Haven Project so far, and Heather said that she has started collecting baseline information from them.

Heather asked whether the next Haven leaflet to be produced should be on self-harm, and aimed at both self-harmers and those who don't understand it. It was suggested that it may be a good idea to give a supply of the leaflets to Colchester A&E Department. The group is interested in working together to compile the self-harm leaflet. In the current draft of the acceptable behaviour policy, self-harm will be classed as unacceptable while present at The Haven. Obviously this is a very sensitive subject and is open to much discussion.

For the questionnaire design for the research, we discussed how we will measure improvement. It should be measured not just from the baseline data, but also from self-reporting and individually tailored care plans. We need to try to capture the identified reasons why; the safety of the atmosphere – how safe is it, what is the continuity doing, how well do the long-term individual tailored care plans work? We agreed that we will need to find a way to measure the tiniest of shifts in changes in each person's life. A possible problem that we may encounter could be the sense of identity in the sickness role, the 'fear of being well'. We talked about identifying the journey of response to inadequate care-givers, that is, has the perception changed towards the care-giver in terms of less expectation and more balanced perceptions? The questions that we will be using in the questionnaire will need to be with the ethics committee by November/December of this year. This means that we need to start putting the questions together at the next meeting. The questionnaire needs to encompass many aspects of the inner and outer world of the individual and will hopefully measure the spectrum from small shifts to significant changes.

Friday 8 October 2004

We are meeting after a three-month break during summer holidays, while setting up the service, and four people attended today. The project has been extremely busy what with the impending visit from the Department of Health and the Guardian newspaper both coming up next week. There have also been some problems with planning issues around our proposed permanent accommodation at Glen Avenue. As a result of this the leaflet concerning self-harm has not been prepared. Heather will draft something up and bring it to the next meeting for discussion.

Heather also mentioned that recruitment for the crisis service staff is now complete and that we have some really good people coming on board. Fifty clients have already registered and it feels like more people are needed to attend the research meetings. We need to approach more people to see if they would be interested in coming on board. Client researchers will be paid for every questionnaire that they complete, the amount to fall within the therapeutic earnings limit. *Boris* was concerned that the groups and activities should also be available in the evenings and at weekends to enable clients who work to have access.

The research questionnaire will not be ready for the ethics committee until January or February of next year now. It has been agreed by the research group that the project needs to have been up and running for many months before the questionnaire can be implemented. This will also allow for things to settle a little after the upheaval of moving premises and all of the new staff coming on board. The group agreed to start to consider questions for the questionnaire and to bring them to next month's meeting.

211

Tuesday 9 November 2004

There are six people attending today with some new members joining the group. The group worked on the draft of the self-harm leaflet which will now be sent out to the whole client mailing list for comment.

The safe centre opened yesterday and four people had used the service last night, all went well. The planning proposals for change of use of Glen Avenue are going to the Planning Committee on 18 November; this means that The Haven Project won't be in the new premises until January 2005. This in turn has slowed down the questionnaire process as the whole service needs to be up and running before data can be collected. The purpose of the research questionnaire was revisited and the research group will help to formulate the questions. Both *Jonny* and *Katy* said they have previous experience of research work. The questionnaire will need to be submitted to the ethics committee for approval before data collection can start. The group discussed the type of questions that it was felt would be useful to include, such as sense of self and coping strategies. It was suggested that the opening questions should be quite innocuous, followed by scaling and tick box questions. Finally, it was felt that questions inviting individual comments and exploration should be included towards the end of the questionnaire.

Tuesday 14 December 2004

Five people attending today, with some new members joining the group. *Harry* and *Jonny* recently went down to Richmond for a couple of days to conduct interviews with the staff, clinical supervisors and course convenors involved in the Henderson/Cassel Hospital PD training course. Both enjoyed the experience immensely and we now have two interviewers for our research.

Baseline information is being collected on the registration forms and will be collected again at the annual re-registration. Hopefully we will then be able to see that money is being saved by less/more appropriate use of services by Haven clients.

On the subject of the questionnaire design and our own research, Heather said that we can already see that some people are feeling an improvement. However, the questionnaire is still some months down the line, because clients will need to access all of the upcoming services, such as reflexology, DBT etc. One idea is to have Recovery Service Evaluation groups every two or three months. This idea was well received by all present and it was agreed that the groups would be called service evaluation groups (SEGs). Hopefully the first 'SEG' will be held in February and this is something we can keep doing until we gain ethical permission for our study.

At the last meeting it was agreed that all members would try to think of some possible questions to be used in the questionnaire. This is a list of questions which were brought to the meeting and agreed by all to be useful and relevant:

- Can you say something about the kinds of responses you have received at The Haven when you have been feeling vulnerable or in crisis?

- What has been your experience of some of the groups, activities, one-to-ones and other therapies at The Haven? These therapies could be listed out for people to rate individually.

- How do you feel The Haven helps you personally?

- Are you learning new skills which are helping you to understand and cope better?

- Could you say something about the kinds of coping strategies you have used and whether these have changed?

- Since coming to The Haven, do you feel you spend less time disliking yourself?

- In what ways, if any, do you feel you have changed as a person since attending The Haven?

- Can you say something about hopes, dreams, goals and the future and whether your vision of this has changed since coming to The Haven?

Tuesday 11 January 2005

Seven present today and there seems to be a stable membership of the group occurring. Not everyone is present at every meeting, but it is a membership of 10: Heather C, *Jonny, Boris, Doris, Harry, Cosmic, Calvin, Katy* and *Curtis*.

The project is due to move and open at Glen Avenue on 31 January 2005. Again, it was agreed that carrying out full research questionnaires and interviews was still many months off because of the need to have the project fully up and running, with all parts of the service, before progress and recovery can be assessed in an in-depth way. Therefore, it was decided that the next meeting of the group on 11 February should be a SEG (service evaluation group) and that a wider section of community members should be invited to attend. This group will be run over two hours, with a break, and will explore the questions formulated at the last meeting, as an interim service evaluation.

Tuesday 8 March 2005

Five present today. Last month, as planned, instead of the research group, a SEG was held (service evaluation group held on 8 February). It was very positive and offered a range of constructive criticism and highlighted help and improvements since The Haven opened. There was a lot of honesty and a lot of laughter and it was good that people felt so open about expressing things, despite the tape recorder, which people seemed to forget once the group got going. It was also agreed that this exercise should be repeated three-monthly, the next one being on Tuesday 10 May, and that an hour and a half, with a break, is a good length. The group reviewed the eight SEG questions and agreed that they should all remain the same for the next evaluation meeting, apart from number four which mentions coping skills and was similar to number five, a bit repetitive. It was agreed that this should be changed to:

Q4 Are you learning new skills which are helping you to understand yourself more?

The subject of being paid for participating in the SEG was discussed. Members of the group felt differently about this. It was felt that payment was about being valued, but others felt people might come just to be paid, and that plenty would come if not paid. It was agreed that travel expenses should still be available and that payment on an hourly basis, as therapeutic earnings, should be offered to those in attendance, but not until the end of the meeting. People could then refuse, accept or donate what was paid.

Heather said that one of her research supervisors from the university, Dr Nicola Morant, had suggested that pseudonyms be used at the SEG, so that progress for individual attendees might be seen more clearly over time. The group agreed and a variety of personal, and sometimes very novel, pseudonyms were suggested!

Harry also suggested that it might be a good idea to include another question in the next SEG. This is about possible fears in relation to recovery, that is, is it getting well scary? Why? In what ways is it scary? It would be really appreciated if group members could give this some thought before the next meeting and, if agreed, we can work out the wording.

Tuesday 12 April 2005

The next SEG will be held on the date of our next research meeting, namely, Tuesday 10 May, from 11 am to 12.45 pm, with a 15-minute break. Posters will be sent out and will go on display advertising this.

The suggestion *Harry* made at the last meeting was considered. This involved considering whether we should include an extra question at the SEG about recovery being frightening. Discussion occurred about the fact that it can be scary to think of getting well. There's no real safety net if difficulties return. One can have had difficulties for decades and have experienced, working, suffering, loss, ageing. Also, people get comfortable and changing this can be very scary because it's about the unknown. It's not something you actively seek because of what might be lurking behind the big door. When you have mental health problems there's a real sense of losing time and that there is a big world outside with stigma and discrimination. In relation to recovery, people can feel rushed and have insufficient support. It has a lot to do with the way in which people are supported. It was agreed that a question in relation to this could yield valuable data. *Doris* suggested it should simply be:

Is recovery frightening?

This was agreed.

Tuesday 15 June 2005

Only three people at the meeting today but 12 people attended the first SEG in February and thirteen the second SEG in May. Although the whole community is invited, this was still considered a good turnout. It was felt that one client tended to dominate the last SEG, in places. It is hoped that we can have the same people, and more, attend the next SEG in August. It was felt that looking back at what was said, in the transcript, helps us to understand ourselves as a community. It's about ownership and having an input. The new question, about recovery being frightening, was felt to be fruitful. It was agreed that topics for the next meeting should be whether the SEG questions stand as they are or whether they should be amended and/or added to. Hopefully there will be more members at the next meeting at the new time of Wednesday afternoons.

Further discussion also occurred about what happens after The Haven, again relating to fears about recovery and the need for a continued safety net.

Wednesday 27 July 2005

A decision needed to be made about the format of the next SEG on 24 August. It was agreed that the same questions should be used and kept as a yardstick. One additional question was suggested:

What else do you feel The Haven could do to support your recovery?

It was agreed that this should be added. This will mean that five questions will have to be answered in the first half and five in the second half.

Invitations to several other clients had been given for them to join us at the research group and it is hoped that they and existing members will be able to make our new time of the last Wednesday afternoon in the month. The next meeting is the SEG and a good attendance is anticipated.

Wednesday 27 September 2005

The last SEG was held on 24 August and it was agreed that this was a very good meeting, real positive movement and a marked difference between those who have been at The Haven for a while and those who have registered more recently. It was also noted that newer people still contributed well at the SEG. This was good because it can take a long time to speak up and trust. It was agreed that the questions for the next SEG on 23 November should remain the same, but this decision has been kept open for research group members who are not present today. However, one reason it is probably good to keep questions the same is that consistent comparisons can be made over time.

The group was made aware of the collection of base line information for our first 25 clients who have been with us a year, showing big drops in annual use of many services including hospital admissions and Sec 136s.

The October meeting is due to fall during Heather C's next study leave week when she will be working on project research, Heather asked if the group would agree to cancel this meeting, but that members could get in touch about anything pertinent before the next SEG. This was agreed.

Tuesday 25 January 2006

We have a new member of the research group, *Rose*, as we have lost one member to an unacceptable behaviour ban.

The fourth SEG was held on 23 November, 2005. The Group felt that, although it was challenging in parts, some very valuable data was captured in relation to recovery. This was around statements from attendees regarding wanting to be challenged in their comfort zone. This is being responded to by the new Progress Planning system at the project, where staff meets to work out a team formulation for individual clients then works with the client to create a long-term, recovery oriented care plan. The next SEG will be held in February this year.

Heather C informed the group that, at last, the research proposal for The Haven had now been submitted to Anglia Ruskin University and was also just about to go to the University Ethics Committee for approval. A copy of the final proposal was given out, together with copies of the information sheet and the consent form for the study. Discussion occurred about preliminary steps to ensure Haven clients are fully aware of the particular part of the study they are taking part in, including having help to read the Information Sheet if they have literacy or dyslexia problems and it also being made clear to such clients that they don't have to read anything as part of the study, questions will be asked rather than having to be read. Once approval has been gained, the SEGs will become focus groups throughout 2006. It was felt that, once the systematic part of the research has been competed, SEGs should still continue in future years, probably continuing every three months, because they have been so valuable to the development of the project. A suggestion had been made by one of Heather C's university supervisors, that we might add to or amend the questions developed. The group felt quite strongly that there are enough questions for an hour and a half and that they would like the same questions to remain as they will be consistent with the SEGs that have already taken place. *Harry* emphasized the need to involve the carers and ideas for carers questions were discussed by the group. These will be suggested to, and refined by, a small number of carers so that they can be used for the two carers' focus groups to be held this year.

216

- What should carers be called? Clients don't always like the term carers as it suggest dependency and something like 'supporters' might be better. This is a key question for the carers to discuss we felt.

- How can carers best be helped? *Harry* said her husband favoured informal support when he needed it, rather than the idea of a supporters group. What support do they feel they personally need? The Henderson workshop for clients and their significant others had been a great success last year and perhaps these kinds of forums might be repeated. This was educational, which highlights the question of information and education and what do carers feel they need in this respect?

- In what ways do carers feel The Haven has helped?

- Is there any more The Haven can do to help?

- Issues around helplessness, especially at times of relapse. Do carers feel hopeless/helpless? Do they have a sense of guilt and frustration? Sometimes overdoses occur when the carer is asleep and it must be pretty awful to awake and find out what's happened. The Haven engenders hope for clients because of its underpinning recovery ethos. But carers are not necessarily given this kind of hope and can feel quite excluded by The Haven. Although we are not always able to give a full picture, because of confidentiality issues, carers need information about what we're doing here.

- Meetings with clients and carers should happen more often if the client gives permission. Some of them haven't even been to The Haven and it was felt that clients sometimes take home a very negative view of how they are and how they are progressing and the carers need to hear more of the positive.

- What does a carer feel recovery is? It might be a totally different concept from that of the client. They might be expecting some magic wand cure. It was also felt that client and carer can become locked into a negative dynamic – dependent/helpless client and rescuer carer. If this is not clearly understood by both parties a carer may unwittingly sabotage progress. *Cosmic* suggested information from Eric Berne's *The Games People Play* and this could possibly be the subject of a workshop for both clients and carers and it would be about a new contract being negotiated between client and carer as recovery progresses.

Individual interviews for clients have also been suggested by university supervisors. The group felt that this could enable us to involve some clients who might not come to a focus group and that people might say things in an interview that they might not say at a group. Interviews would ideally be carried out by a client. It was agreed by all present that *Jonny* should carry out the interviews to be done in the first part of 2006. Apart from being an experienced researcher, she has also never used Haven crisis services and this would, hopefully, present less of a boundary issue for clients. It may be that other members are further along in their progress and can become involved in the follow-up interviews which will occur at a later date. The importance of stressing that people should feel comfortable with the person interviewing them was discussed. This is covered in information and consent forms, giving the right to withdraw at any stage.

The group questioned whether other information gathered from clients will be used, like base line information of use of services and other questionnaires for the national evaluation. Heather C felt that all this data could be used as background to the study.

Tuesday 26 April 2006

The February meeting was a SEG on 22 February, and the next Research Meeting, due to be held on 22 March was cancelled due to staffing shortages. The fifth SEG held in February was excellent with some real shifts apparent for some people.

The Haven internal research and Heather's PhD have fallen by the wayside this year, due to the staffing difficulties and pressures. The question this afternoon is, can it be salvaged? *Jonny* and *Doris* felt that it must be and Heather C said she had spoken to the Service Manager who says she is keen to cover study weeks for Heather C to enable this to happen.

Heather C said that her supervisors, Shula and Nicola, had both suggested that the SEG questions need some adjustment before focus groups can be held. *Doris* felt it was important not to lose the current questions but that we should be open to smaller tweaks and suggestions, especially in relation to recovery-type questions. A discussion occurred about the simplicities and the subtleties of recovery, namely, being able to go into town is your short-term goal and you manage to go in and do your shopping – that's a first step – it's all about steps. Also, you can get to the finishing line and slip back. It's all about steps and reaching plateaus. *Jonny* said one very notable thing was that when people at the project are going down now they are picking up a lot quicker.

Heather said there wouldn't be a research meeting before the next SEG and we probably wouldn't be at the stage of modifying the questions, and getting ethical approval, and being able to run it as a focus group. She also said that Shula had mentioned that external supervisors were talking about the possible need for independent facilitation of the focus groups. *Jonny* and *Boris* agreed with Heather that this is collaborative research and that the clients don't hold back in relation to what they say at SEGs because Heather is facilitating – quite the contrary sometimes! It was noted that clients involved in the national evaluation's individual interviews and focus group, in March, presented a glowing picture of the project all round and perhaps weren't as honest with outsiders as they are at the SEGs. However, discussion also occurred about it being important to prove a lack of bias in the study and it was agreed that *Jonny* would facilitate the focus groups as well as the interviews. Heather said she hoped to talk to her supervisors to see what they were looking at in terms of question modifications but that she felt the research timetable realistically needed to be extended. It was agreed that this would make more sense if data collection took place until mid-2007, rather than stopping in February 2007.

It would be possible to carry out the proposed carers' focus groups in this timescale and the research group had already begun suggestions for the carers at the last meeting. What Heather needs to do is to hold a meeting with some of the carers to also get their input regarding possible questions. This needs to be done soon.

The individual interviews pose a trickier problem. Now that we are only registering two clients a month it is much harder to get 20 interviews 'before' and 20 interviews 'after'. It was felt that a much better idea would be to capture the before/after aspects within the interview questions themselves and look at a more comprehensive interview schedule than for the SEGs/focus groups, namely, mapping the journey of recovery. *Jonny* is still keen to do the individual interviews and it would be ideal if these could begin in June and could target a range/variety of clients. The national evaluators also aimed at a variety of clients in terms of gender, circumstances, age, time at project, use of services etc. It was felt that the right interview schedule, for the individual interviews, could capture the journey in an exciting way with all its 'speed bumps' and detours.

Heather said that, although her research proposal had been approved, the timescales are not as above and she wasn't sure how this would link up with the Ethics Committee application. She also said Shula had asked her to contact the National Evaluation to see how much of their data can be shared. Heather has done so and this will be possible and an interim report will be available in the next couple of months.

Wednesday 28 June 2006

The May meeting was a SEG. The May SEG transcript has been ready for over two weeks but Heather C hasn't had an opportunity to check it. It should be distributed to the research group and SEG attendees very soon.

Near to final drafts of focus group questions and the interview questionnaire had been circulated in recent weeks. Heather C said she had reviewed the drafts with Shula and Nicola yesterday and the group now needed to make some final decisions to enable a submission to the University Ethics Committee for permission to carry out the research:

219

- Carer focus group questions: This had been circulated to five carers and concern was expressed about question four, 'Do you experience personal difficulties regarding the person you support? If yes, can you say something about these difficulties?' Even though results are anonymized, some carers felt that they would be reticent to say anything about who they support. Heather C had suggested making it more general like, 'Do you think carers experience… etc.' Shula had alternatively suggested, 'Research shows that carers often experience difficulties in caring. Do you think this statement is correct and, if so, in what way do you think the role affects carers?' This was unanimously agreed as the new question four. Shula had also suggested that every group and interview should end with, 'Have you got anything more to add?' Again this was agreed for focus groups and the interviews. Heather C said that Toni, who is a carer for a Haven client, had agreed to facilitate the carer focus groups and members agreed this was a good choice.

- Client focus group questions: The latest draft of the client focus group questions was discussed. The altered sequence of some of the questions, and the more open-ended wording was agreed. The new question four about community was also agreed. Nicola's suggested amendment to question five, namely, '…what do you gain from these new skills?' was agreed. However the suggestion that question six should change to, 'Since coming to The Haven have you changed the way you feel about yourself?' was rejected and members still want to keep, 'Since coming to The Haven do you feel you spend less time disliking yourself?' because somehow this way of phrasing seems to speak to PD.

- Client interview: The questions on page two will be consistent with the changes discussed for the client focus group questionnaire above. There are also an additional two questions, one about how The Haven compares with other services, and another one about community which asks about interaction and support between clients. Both additions were agreed and it was noted that there will be more time to ask questions during the individual interviews. *Jonny* focused our attention on getting the individual interviews started and felt there should be an introductory paragraph to guide her and the respondent into the interview. *Nicola* had suggested that actual age is included, not just age range. It was pointed out that marital status should also include civil partnership as well as married/living as. Additional questions at the end of page one were agreed, namely, 'How long have you been using the project?' and also additional boxes about which parts of the service are being used by the respondent.

Jonny was asked to outline her research experience for the application form because she will be conducting the major part of groups and interviews. Apart from her involvement in the Henderson/Cassel PD course research last year, she has also carried out research in the past in education, social care, and animal behaviour and ecology. It looks like we are now ready to go to Ethics Committee and the next SEG will hopefully be a client focus group. It is hoped that the first carer focus group will happen in August, or soon after, and that the individual interviews will start soon after that.

Wednesday 27 September 2006

The last meeting in July was just *Jonny* and Heather C and we discussed the application for ethical permission and the next stage of the research. No minutes were distributed.

The research proposal received permission from Anglia Ruskin University in March this year, and ethical permission to carry out the research was granted by the University Ethics Committee in August.

We have already held six SEGs with lots of relevant data. The first client focus group was held in August and the transcript will be ready soon. *Jonny* facilitated this and has also carried out the first Individual client interview. Her aim is to get something like two interviews done per month. The next client focus group is on 22 November. We are aiming to have the first carer focus group in October or November, facilitated by Toni. This may have to be held during an evening. There were lots of suggested people for individual interviewees, most of who don't usually come to SEGs/focus groups. Twenty were suggested in all, 8 men and 12 women, with a good range including younger and older members, and single, divorced, parents, etc.

The group discussed the idea of a transitional recovery category at The Haven which would be a category that people who were really making progress in their recovery could graduate to with pride. However, we looked at all the systems that will need to be in place to achieve this, in addition to the crisis and therapeutic input The Haven gives. The study and work peer support group needs support and there is also a whole spectrum of educational needs from confidence to literacy. Voluntary work, as a good introduction to eventual paid work, was discussed, plus the idea of clients going in two's and three's initially. It was agreed that, in order to successfully map the Journey of Recovery in the research, it would be necessary for The Haven to have a full spectrum of support and skills available to its clients.

Wednesday 28 March 2007

We have two new members of the group, *Jenny* and *Poppy*, and a good turnout today. It was noted that this is the first meeting of the research group this year. The purpose of the meeting is to take stock of what data we have collected so far, and what data we still have to collect between now and July. It is also important to begin to think of categories, themes, or codes, for the research data, to enable it to be separated out for analysis.

221

Data collected so far:

SEGs (Service Evaluation Groups) – *informal data*

6 groups 2005/2006 = approx 180 pages

Client focus groups – *formal data*

3 groups 2006/2007 = approx 100 pages

Care Focus Group – *formal data*

1 group 2007 + approx 40 pages

Client Individual Interviews – *formal data*

13 interviews 2006/2007 + approx 280 pages

Total = approx **600 pages** of verbatim transcripts

Additional informal data

Research Group Minutes

Advisory Group Minutes

Minutes of Discussions

Newsletter

Creative Writing

Still to be collected:

Client focus group – formal data

1 group = approx 30 pages

Care focus group – formal data

1 group = approx 30 pages

Client individual interviews – formal data

7 interviews = approx 140 pages

Grand total = approx 800 pages

It was agreed that this is a vast amount of data and we need to begin thinking of ideas for categories and themes that seem to be emerging and which relate to recovery in personality disorder and The Haven. Following is a list of initial ideas from the group.

Initial ideas for themes emerging:

Safety

Issues of trust

Boundaries and boundary testing

Betrayals

Loss of trust

Misconceptions about recovery

What is recovery?

Hope

Fear of failure

The importance of peer support

What were the main coping strategies?

How did people feel about themselves to begin with?

Shedding old coping strategies

The pain of trying to move on

Split/dichotomy – their fault/my fault – blame

Letting go of the past

Losing idea of how family was, or even losing family

Loss and grieving process

Blips and relapses

Faster recovery from blips with insight

Changing sense of self

New messages about self from Haven community

Internalising new messages/good ideas about self

Being and feeling valued

Valuing self and others

The community as home and parent

Power sharing and feeling in control

Being trusted with responsibility

Being recognized for skills

Comparisons with other services

Recovery comes from person themselves

It's not all down to The Haven

The Haven is life saver vs. The Haven is too safe and holds you back

Stuck in learned helplessness	Rewarding constructiveness and progress
The response to learned helplessness is tough love	Small steps
	Developmental process, learning to walk, leaving 'parents'/Haven
	Fear of loss of support
	Fear of failure
	Sense of identity when recovering – who am I, where am I, where do I fit in?
	The concept of transitional recovery/ need for safety net/secure attachment
	A new set of trust issues – with the outside world
	Huge issue of benefits and money – basic survival
	Wanting to work and being given a chance
	Realizing that recovery is an onward journey for everyone

223

Wednesday 25 April 2007

The fourth and last client focus group will be next month, on 23 May. The date for the second carer focus group needs to be set for July. Thirteen individual client interviews are complete and there are seven still to do. A discussion occurred about who might be included in the seven and how we can keep a balance of gender and other factors. It was also agreed that two people who were no longer at the project, due to unacceptable behaviour, should be approached as this could give an interesting dimension to the data being collected.

Although the meeting next month will be a client focus group, the next Research Group meeting will be on Wednesday 27 June from 2 pm to 3 pm. It is now very important that we have good attendance at research meetings to enable us to work together on analysis of the findings.

Wednesday 27 June 2007

We have now held the fourth and last client focus group. A decision needs to be made on whether, in two months' time, to have an SEG in August. It was agreed, yes, because why change a successful action and it will also give more background data to the research. The second and last carer focus group will be in July (now 3 August). Sixteen individual interviews have been done so far, four men and

12 women, which follows project ratio of clients. Consideration was also given to age and status in terms of children, married or single, etc. and we have been fairly inclusive so far. Five names were suggested, four of whom will be selected to complete the 20.

It remains important that we have good attendance at research meetings to enable us to work together on analysis of the findings.

Wednesday 25 July 2007

Heather C had not had a chance to look at the transcript for the fourth, and last, client focus group, which will be sent out to everyone soon. The second and last carer focus group will be held on 3 August, with time afterwards for carers to talk together informally – the first families and carers group? Nineteen out of the 20 individual client interviews are done and discussion occurred about who the last participant should be. So far *Jonny* has interviewed 14 women and five men. Age ranges are quite well spread over younger, middle, older. Home conditions in terms of having a partner, children, or not, are also quite well spread. Twelve clients were considered, with three being most desirable. One will be interviewed over the next week. This will be the end of data collection and Heather C thanked members of the group who have attended recently as we move into the phase of data analysis.

Wednesday 26 September 2007

Only three of us were attending today, *Jonny*, *Poppy* and Heather C. All data is now collected, however, Heather C's next study leave is not until the end of October. This is when data analysis will begin. For this reason it was decided to cancel the October meeting until some preliminary data analysis has been completed to enable this to be brought back to the research group. The meeting took a look again at the categories that had been suggested at the March meeting, earlier this year, and this mapping of the recovery process will be taken into account when Heather C begins the analysis.

A SEG was held on 24 August and the transcript from this will be made available in coming weeks. The next research group meeting would fall during the Christmas holidays, therefore, it was decided that a meeting may need to be scheduled before then as initial comments will be needed on data analysis. Heather C will consult with members about this.

Wednesday 30 January 2008

A good turnout today with most members of the group here, including *Calvin* who is back. It is our first meeting since September and Toni has joined us in relation to the data from family members and carer focus groups and members were happy to have her present.

Poppy and *Cosmic*, although unable to make today's meeting, have both agreed to help with data analysis, detailed below.

In November a SEG was held. Again, in December, it was agreed that data analysis needed to progress and Heather C had study leave in January and good progress is now been made on the analysis.

Originally we held SEGs (service evaluation groups) every three months and six were held over a year and a half. These turned into four focus groups held over one year. Since then we have resumed the SEGs at three-monthly intervals and two have been held. Heather C said that, in research terms, she feels we have reached saturation point for data collection. However, the SEGs serve an important function in themselves in that they continue to give client feedback for monitoring project progress, and they give new clients an opportunity to feed back in a structured way. *Harry* suggested that, once data analysis is complete, we resume the SEGs on a six-monthly basis. This was agreed. We also discussed the idea of follow-up feedback being invited from research participants. As we know, since focus groups and individual interviews took place, some clients have made significant further progress. Some may also have had setbacks and have bounced back from these. It was felt that it could be important to capture developments and progress for individuals as part of the findings. It was also suggested that carers and family members should be included in any invitations to send in more data.

Heather C said that we have 770 pages of data! It was agreed that it is a good thing that so many people want to help. It was also agreed that ten clients and a carer involved in data analysis will really be in the spirit of our research which is *participatory* action research. The data collected is as follows:

Table A2.1 Data collected

6 SEGs Feb 05 to May 06	Informal data
4 Client focus groups Aug 06 to May 07	Formal data
20 Client individual interviews Aug 06 to Aug 07	Formal data
2 Carer focus groups March 07 and Aug 07	Formal data
2 SEGs Aug 07 and Nov 07	Informal data

During her study leave this month Heather C had coded all 770 pages manually, she had marked, with different coloured pens, 14 categories detailed below which we will eventually narrow down to some of the themes discussed at our March meeting. She then used a computer program called NVivo7 to begin to put all the quotes she had coded together in one place. During study leave she had managed to do this only for the first category, trust and safety. She had spent 17 hours last weekend trying to complete the rest but had only managed to get two-thirds done, but hoped to complete everything this weekend so that transcripts were available to the group. She said that, although there are 14 different categories so far, she suggested keep in mind three areas that seem to speak to respondents in terms of recovery, namely, dependence on psychiatric services, psychological changes, and social progress.

Table A 2.2 Three recovery issues

1	Am I able to cope with less support in terms of hospital admissions?
2	Am I feeling better, symptomatology, able to see the future, etc?
3	Do I feel valued in terms of my contributions in life/social inclusion?

It was decided that different group members would take responsibility for reading through different categories. Some transcripts are much larger than others and quotes collected for each category so far were given to the group. Below is a list of each category and how many pages each transcript turned out to be.

Table A2.3 Categories for client research group members to work on

Number	Category	Pages
1	Trust: Safety: Consistency: Responsiveness	37
2	The community	51
3	Empowerment: Confidence	18
4	Service savings: Changing coping strategies	79
5	Feeling cared for	9
6	Non-judgement: Respect	9
7	Self-worth	35
8	Hope: Recovery: Social inclusion	132
9	Being challenged	11
10	Attachment	4
	Categories for Toni to work on	
11	The term carer	4
12	Burden: Guilt	20
13	Involving and supporting carers and family	9
	Needs more work by Heather C	
14	Service developments	

This last category is about research affecting the development of The Haven and, although coding has been done through all 770 pages, this needs more reflection. Although quotes from the carer focus groups are included in some of the first ten categories, identity is protected. However, it was felt that the more sensitive aspects of that data, for example, 'Burden: Guilt', should be further analyzed by Toni because of confidentiality issues.

The transcripts were assigned as follows:

Table A2.4 Transcript categories

Number	Category	Primary	Secondary
1	Trust: Safety: Consistency: Responsiveness	*Boris*	*Jonny*
2	The community	*Doris*	
3	Empowerment: Confidence	*Harry*	
4	Service Savings: Changing coping strategies	*Curtis*	
5	Feeling cared for	*Poppy*	
6	Non-judgement: Respect	*Calvin*	*Katy*
7	Self-worth	*Katy*	*Rose*
8	Hope: Recovery: Social inclusion	*Jonny*	*Harry*
9	Being challenged	*Cosmic*	*Doris*
10	Attachment	*Rose*	*Boris*
11	The term carer	*Toni*	
12	Burden: Guilt	*Toni*	
13	Involving and supporting carers and family	*Toni*	

Some people have agreed to read through a second category and comments on both your choices will be welcome. Comments will be needed from the primary list by the next research group meeting, date below. Guidelines as follows:

1. Read through full transcript and note if anything is in there that you feel shouldn't be.

2. Reflect on what this category is telling us.

3. Are there further categories within this category, i.e. can it be broken down further, for example, hope, recovery and social inclusion is huge and will definitely need to be broken down, as will some of the others.

4. Are there categories that you feel should be in there that aren't?

5. Anything else you would like to add?

It was noted that Heather C had spotted some mistakes in transcription which she had missed. In focus Group 3, in some places *Norris* should be *Boris* and this needs changing. In one transcript *Rose* says she's given up cannabis! This has definitely been changed to *Ruth* has given it up!! We also have two people called *Sally* and the one from the individual client interview is shown as *Sally 2* in the categories. We also have *Emma* as a pseudonym and this will need to be changed in due course as it is the actual name of one of our clients.

What we are doing here is just a beginning in mapping the journey of recovery in PD from this data. It will need to be broken down and then refined during the year into the major themes. A full analysis of service developments in relation to the research will also need to be done. Further categorization, by client, will also occur, that is, all the bits from *Harry, Boris* and for every participant throughout the data will be drawn together. This is where the invitation for follow-up data could be valuable, to complete any case history type results we want to present. Heather C said that research supervisors were also stressing that it will be important to show, in the results, the reflective journey of this group.

Wednesday February 27 2008

Jonny had taken on the largest category 'Hope, recovery and social inclusion' which is 132 pages and definitely needs to be broken down into smaller categories. She had managed to get through 39 pages so far and felt that the further categories should break down into 'Hope', 'Recovery', 'Changing attitudes' and 'Social inclusion'. She also suggested a further break-down into negative and positive responses in the categories. Heather C said that supervisors at the university had also suggested this. *Jonny's* notes on the first 39 pages also reflected other issues, for example, drawing out the spectrum of recovery and social inclusion issues, not just employment; issues about respect; being challenged; fear of change and its relationship to attachment; the strong link between recovery and trust, and perfectionism and their relationship to unrealistic goals and aims and how this is a hard nut to crack.

Doris had looked at the category 'Being challenged' which is 11 pages, and felt this could be broken down into 'Dealing with challenging behaviour' and 'Being challenged/pushed'. She felt that 'Challenging behaviour' might best be in the 'Community' section. Heather C said that quotes about 'Challenging behaviour' had also been included in the 'Community' category. *Doris* has 'Community' as her main category and hasn't made a start on this yet – it is another big one at 51 pages.

Rose had taken on 'Attachment' which is four pages. Her analysis reflected on the sense of family at The Haven in relation to attachment; the fact that community is a safety net; the fear of losing The Haven being tied to the fear of recovery; the issue of learning to trust being related to being able to ask for help; non-judgement and acceptance as part of attachment that helped people to stand on their own two feet; the importance of nurturing attachment so that there is no pushing for discharge; the fact that the carers focus group also felt the staff were friends; that The Haven represented a home but that this was also hard for family to accept; that carers too wanted The Haven to be around forever and their biggest worry is loss of The Haven for their family member; carers also reflected on whether, if The Haven is working for them, their family member would have to move on and fears from the carer/family member that other people might think their family member didn't need The Haven; in relation to clients again there was a sense of being checked-up on and being cared for and being able to come in at any time; that clients wondered how quickly you would get support back from The Haven if they made progress but then relapsed; and finally that for many clients The Haven becomes the family they have lost or never had.

Poppy had taken on 'Feeling cared for' which is nine pages. She wanted to do more work on it but so far she felt that it was highlighting issues such as feeling wanted; belonging, how you are greeted at the door; whether you are let down; and the importance of pampering and complementary therapies which involve touch and are nurturing.

Toni had taken on the carer focus group categories of 'The term carer' which is four pages, 'Burden and guilt' which is 20 pages, and 'Involving and supporting carers and family' which is nine pages. She said that 'The term carer' had shown that 'carer' is a contentious issue and a double-edged term. In one way it is a known term that is recognized by statutory agencies including social services and welfare benefits agencies but that family members can feel that it is patronising, not to mention the service user, and it doesn't really describe who they are, which may be husband or wife, etc. Toni said she needed to do more work on 'Burden and guilt' and didn't feedback at the meeting on this category. On 'Involving and supporting carers and family' it was interesting that some carers/family members didn't want to be involved and definitely saw The Haven as their family member's place and did not want to destroy any trust between Haven and client, which was quite perceptive. The carers/family members seemed very aware of the delicate situation of whether they should ring and whether their significant-other would want them to have information.

Others hadn't done a lot as yet on their categories. *Calvin* is working on 'Non-judgement and respect' with Toni. *Curtis* needs to start on 'Service savings and changing coping strategies'. Heather C said that supervisors at the university had pointed out that this category was wrongly named in that service users would not be focusing on 'service savings'. This is, however, relevant to funders and could be included in a chapter analysing results, but it should not be the name of a category. Everyone agreed with this and the name of the category will be changed. *Boris* had not made a start on 'Trust, safety, consistency and responsiveness'. *Harry* on 'Empowerment and confidence building', *Katy* on 'Self-worth' and *Cosmic* on 'Being challenged' weren't at the meeting today and there hasn't been any feedback from them yet.

Heather C said that university supervisors had suggested that we might want to do some work as a group on analysing some of this so it was agreed to spend the second half of the meeting, the remaining half hour, analysing 'Empowerment and confidence' together. We did this but only got through 4½ pages out of 19 in the half hour. So, it is a very slow job. Issues we noted included the fact that the choice to attend is empowering; empowerment links to trust; empowerment links to caring and being able to give as well as take; setting goals can be empowering and even if you are feeling bad you can maintain some confidence; empowerment is learning from each other; the sense of ownership at The Haven is empowering and the fact that clients are able to affect and control things; learning to speak up in groups is both learning to trust and confidence building; being believed in and trusted can give you confidence outside and even to start work; insight and self-management is empowering; encouragement to reflect is empowering because it throws the issue back on self; helping others increased self-knowledge and self-worth; internalizing positive comments from others can increase confidence; support without being taken over helps you to help yourself; pushing yourself even when you don't want to is a sign of confidence; being able to speak out at conferences shows a big leap in confidence; having people behind you gives you courage; having been brave enough to challenge staff and see that the relationship held-up increases trust and confidence; gaining confidence in groups at The Haven gives confidence to join groups outside; confidence relates to non-judgement, acceptance and trust.

Wednesday 26 March 2008

Reflecting on data analysis, there was a discussion about the importance of a follow-up for certain clients who have been very involved in Haven research, especially if they are going to be sited as case studies. It was agreed that Heather C should code all data for each individual client involved in the research into individual transcripts.

Again, the importance of reinstituting the SEGs, once data analysis is complete, was agreed. *Harry* and *Jonny* stressed that this was important not just for ongoing service evaluation of the project, but also to give new clients the same sense of ownership and belonging that had been generated for clients who had been here longer.

The rest of the meeting was spent in a continued analysis of the category 'Empowerment and confidence'.

Wednesday 30 April 2008

Heather C said she had used her last study leave week, earlier this month, to bring together individual data for the 60 clients involved in Haven research. She brought the 60 transcripts to the meeting and group members now have a copy of their individual transcripts.

Some Haven clients just attended one focus group, SEG or individual interview, however, some people have data from many meetings and individual interviews and this represents two and a half years of data for that person. It is possible to see clear patterns of improvement, over time, for many people. Heather will be using her study leave week in August to analyze the transcripts further in terms of how many men and how many women, age groups, and responses to particular questions, for example on a preliminary look at the data, for questions like, *'Since coming to The Haven do you spend less time disliking yourself?'*, it seems that there is a pattern of improvement to responses after a period of six months. These are the kinds of patterns and themes we'll be looking for in the individual data. Members agreed to read their own transcripts and feedback.

We are also continuing with analysis of themes as follows:

Jonny and Boris – 'Trust'

Harry to finish 2nd half of 'Confidence and empowerment'

Katy is half way through 'Self-worth'

Poppy is part way through 'Feeling cared for'

Jonny wants to look at breaking down 'Hope, recovery and social inclusion'

Rose will have a go at 'Non-judgement and respect'

Wednesday 28 May 2008

Incomplete tasks were reassigned as follows:

Jonny and *Katy* – 'Trust'

Doris to do 'Community'

Katy has finished 'Self-worth'

Poppy will finish 'Feeling cared for'

Rose: 'Non-judgement and respect'

Jonny and Heather C 'Hope, recovery and social inclusion'.

Otherwise, people agreed to read their own transcripts as most members of the group had not done so yet.

Wednesday 25 June 2008

Rose gave notes on her analysis of 'Non-judgement and respect'. Remaining tasks are in progress.

Some people had now read their own transcripts of all research events brought together and could really see progress over time.

Wednesday 27 August 2008

Harry has resigned from the research group due to time commitments for her postgraduate course. *Harry* was thanked for her valuable contributions to The Haven research over the past four years.

Heather C reported about her recent week's study leave. She said she had gone through all 60 individual interview transcripts again to draw out responses to the various questions. This had taken some days and had caused her to come to the conclusion that we can't skip over a presentation of the data in terms of the individual research questions and concentrate only on the analysis of themes. She felt that there had been a reluctance to do this, since data collection ended last November, not just because 60 clients were involved, but because many clients answered the questions more than once, multiple times for some, at different research events. The questions also changed sequence over time and some were only asked to those clients individually interviewed. It is a simply massive job, but it must be done. A lot of her week's study leave was spent working out a template for easier access to data on each question for each individual, and the first four questions are now done. A transcript was made available at the meeting, beginning with numerical tables, and data on the four questions.

Heather C said she didn't want people to feel they had wasted time on the analysis of themes, because this crucial data comes later, and work should continue on it. However, there is no way that the questions-analysis can wait until Heather C's next study leave in December. She said that research supervisors had been saying, for some time, that the analysis needs more time, and she intends to work out with day staff a number of individual days, between now and December, to get the client-questions-analysis done.

A timetable was considered, as follows:

1. Research group to read first draft of data analysis and give verbal feedback about credibility at the next meeting at the end of September.

2. Heather C to complete analysis for the remaining ten client questions between now and December.

3. Heather C to complete carers focus group question analysis by the end of the year, which feels like a comparatively tenable task compared to client-question-analysis.

4. Thematic analysis of the 14 themes, including work from this group, to be carried forward in Heather C's December study leave.

5. Several case studies to be considered, as the final section of data, early next year.

There was a discussion about some of the findings in the first four questions, for example, negatives and the importance of The Haven having learned from this feedback. This is relevant in many ways, like 'trust'; what built up trust? What shattered trust? etc.

Consideration was given to what remains on the analysis of themes:

'Trust' – *Jonny* and *Katy* will complete work on this

'Community' – *Doris* would like to see the question-analysis on this first. This is the next question, No. 5, and should be done soon

'Self-worth' – *Katy* to complete

Hope, recovery and social inclusion – *Jonny* is half-way through and will continue.

Wednesday 24 September 2008

The group looked through the timetable now formulated for data analysis:

1. Research group to read first draft of the data analysis and give verbal feedback about credibility at the next meeting.

2. Heather C to complete analysis for the remaining ten clients between now and December.

3. Heather C to complete question analysis by end of the year.

4. Thematic analysis of the themes, including work on the themes from this group, to be carried forward in Heather C's December study leave.

Wednesday 29 October 2008

Feedback from the group, regarding questions one to eight, was that they showed a real indication of progress – how far people have come – and how progress is different for different people – continued movement. People felt that the analysis was definitely now on the right track.

Heather C said that she will be seeing the university research supervisors next week and hasn't yet had feedback from them. How she is feeling now is that the results should form three chapters:

1. *The data* – which will be client questions 1 to 14 (and we are now past the half-way mark) and carer questions from the two focus groups.

2. *Data analysis* – which will include the thematic analysis of the stages of recovery mapped in our research, e.g. Trust and safety, The community and

learning, Confidence and self-esteem, etc. *Jonny* is continuing to work on remaining transcripts with other group members, at the moment, e.g. *Katy*.

3. *Case studies* – this will be a summation and illustration of progress from a few individual perspectives.

Heather C has seven individual days booked for study between now and Christmas and feels she can complete all the question analyses, including carers, during this time. The next meeting of The Haven Research Group will be on Wednesday 28 January 2009 from 2 am to 3 pm. (If there is a need for a meeting before this date it will be called on an ad hoc basis.)

Wednesday 28 January 2009

Our last meeting was in October. The completed preliminary analysis of client questions had already been circulated to the 60 participants, however, since the last meeting the family and carer data has also been analyzed. There were ethical considerations about distributing transcripts to the research group, because family members of some of the group took part, but the research group were very interested to hear about the kinds of responses there had been, and in what numbers. The family and carer transcript has been sent out to the six participants, asking if they would like identity further protected in terms of identifying gender of family member and other factors. None have requested this as yet and, if none do, the research group would feel comfortable about the data being shared more widely.

At the last meeting it had been decided that the data would be presented in three parts. However, supervisors felt that the transcripts of the question analysis were too long to include in the body of the research report and need to go into an appendix. On 6 February Heather C has to send university research supervisors an outline about the next chapters regarding the data. It was agreed that this should be as follows:

1. A précis of the questions analysis which refers back to the appendices.

2. Thematic analysis of the stages of recovery drawing from the work we did last year, picking out the themes that map the process of recovery in PD, i.e. a conceptual map or framework about the logical steps enabling change, grounded into specifics.

3. Case studies – a small number.

4. Discussion about the findings.

A lengthy discussion then took place about issues that had arisen at Heather C's recent tutorial. This included risks in the journey of recovery, current social factors, that is, learned helplessness, fear, and the welfare rights system, all against the background of the current economic crisis affecting employment opportunities.

We discussed whether recovery does occur against the odds and it was agreed that it does – not just the poor odds of a difficult start. Biographical issues were also discussed and simple profiling has been built into the research in terms of age, how long at the project and other daily living data, however, it was felt that some might be willing to have biographical details of trauma included, and others not. There was also a discussion about 'social capital' and the notion that those with better physical health, positive family ties, and better levels of education, might recovery more easily. The group did not feel this was the case with PD where some who fitted this criteria were not progressing well at all, yet others who had been disadvantaged in so many ways continued to progress.

Wednesday 25 March 2009

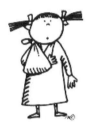

The February meeting had to be cancelled because Heather C fractured her wrist on the way to pick up *Boris* and *Doris* to speak at a conference in Suffolk about developing PD services. While Heather C went to hospital to get 'plastered', *Boris* and *Doris* went to Suffolk and did the conference themselves, to rave reviews. Although she has been hampered by some left-handed typing, Heather C has been continuing with the data analysis.

Heather C had circulated the first two themes of the thematic analysis to the group: *A sense of safety and building trust*; and *Feeling cared for*. She is currently working on the next theme: *A sense of community and belonging*.

These analyses are coming from the themed transcripts compiled last year and the work individual group members carried out on those transcripts, together with work carried out at the group. Some group members had read the analyses so far and some had not. Those who had, felt it was building up in the right way. *Doris* made some interesting comments regarding the physical and mental aspects of being cared for, namely, physical being everything from a cuppa (cup of tea), to a hug, to pampering, being greeted, listening, valuing, etc. Then there was a discussion about the sequence of the remaining themes, and the consensus was that themes involving sense of self/self-worth/self-esteem/confidence should come before recovery and goal oriented themes. This is because the ability to formulate and pursue goals realistically comes from developing self-esteem and confidence, otherwise 'fantasy goals' can present themselves which are unrealistic.

The sequence, after the first three themes above, might be – changing coping strategies, skills, then self-worth, esteem, confidence, and then recovery and goals. It was felt that a later theme should be about healthy attachment and the outside world as this is crucial to understanding recovery in PD. It was agreed that the thematic analysis should remain fluid and open to comment and amendment as we progress.

Heather C said that, last week, she had gone to spend the afternoon with staff from the Norvic Clinic in Norwich which was really fruitful. She had received an email from the team saying that they found The Haven inspirational and uplifting and that it was not all about schema-this and schema-that, but about real people and down to earth solutions. The group felt that this is what we want our research to be human – real language about real people. *Cosmic* suggested this might be called 'PD for Dummies'! (It's already been done *Cosmic*.)

Heather C also made the revamped charts available at the meeting and *Jonny* asked for a copy of these.

Wednesday 27 May 2009

Heather C had circulated a transcript of the first four themes and said she hoped to circulate the whole analysis of themes before the next meeting. *Jonny* had read the first four, but *Cosmic* said he hadn't received it and Heather C had no feedback from anyone else other than a valuable conversation with *Doris* and *Jenny* about barriers to recovery and people becoming defined by the diagnosis and the sick role, so we discussed what had been written up so far. It was agreed that transitional recovery should be the final theme because it's the safety net for the whole journey.

There was a further discussion about the fact that later progress, like being able to be in therapy and contain experiences, and being able to have hope and develop realistic dreams and goals, and achieve things, depended on the earlier building blocks. This wasn't just about building trust and the nice things like being cared for and being part of something, it's also about being able to keep the boundaries or you just don't move forward until those earlier steps are consistently achieved.

Wednesday 24 June 2009

Heather C had circulated the analysis of themes to the research group and it will now be sent to all respondents quoted in it, clients, carers and family members, to share the analysis and ensure accuracy. The group had picked up a couple of typos which will be corrected. Group members thought the analysis was great and felt that the chart/pyramid was a really helpful way to illustrate themes at the beginning of the analysis and that it represents growth and progress.

Incorporating the carer and family data was also of great interest to the group as this had not been made available to them before. Heather C said that university supervisors had made suggestions but generally seemed pleased with progress.

Also, Shula had stressed the importance of highlighting differences about people who are progressing and those who are not. This will be covered in the discussion chapter which will be written next. The group felt that the statements were interesting from some clients who are no longer at The Haven, namely, about it being too late for recovery. The fact that some become stuck in a sickness role was also discussed.

The next important task for the group is to help in the analysis of the research group's function in the research. This will be covered in the updated version of the Methodology chapter, and the group's input and experiences will be central to this. *Jonny's* experiences will be very important as the principle interviewer. It was agreed that the group will not meet in July due to the 5th birthday celebrations at The Haven on that day, but would meet for the August and September meetings. At these meetings, the group will focus on its own processes during the course of the research.

A letter had been sent before this meeting to say that, if members did not give apologies about their non-attendance, we would assume that they did not wish to continue. It was agreed that this should be considered to be the case for *Curtis* who seems to have stopped coming for quite a while. In a few months a further decision will need to be made about whether the group continues in some form or disbands, that is, whether further research will be considered or not, in addition to the re-introduction of the SEG every six months. *Jonny* has been keen for a twin study to be carried out as a very high percentage of Haven clients appear to be one of a pair of twins.

237

Wednesday 26 August 2009

As agreed at the last meeting, the purpose of this meeting and our meeting in September will be to look at what it has meant for participants to be members of the Research Group.

Jonny: Being involved in the research group has led to so much for me, including now doing research for other universities, even Greenwich University now. It's increased my confidence, sense of purpose and I have also been paid. The overall feeling of influencing the minds of professionals with the results our research has yielded. Also, the privilege of getting the vote of confidence from everyone to do the interviews and facilitate the focus groups, to be trusted was a privilege. This has led to other things and when I give input at talks and meetings it gets a really good response and I'm told, 'We don't get this in other lectures.'

Rose: First of all, being part of the SEGs, I learned that we were really being listened to and I actually saw the changes being made in response to what we said. Being part of this research group and seeing it all come together and knowing I've been a part of it and that things have moved on in a measurable way. I'm beginning to get there with a bit more confidence and self-esteem.

Calvin: People found their voices because of the research, where they hadn't found them before. Things have changed in the last ten years and that's been partially to do with this group and also to do with the earlier research group that I was involved in, before The Haven. Being part of these research groups is being actively involved in making changes, including when I was part of the National Group.

It was agreed that we need to try to get feedback from *Boris, Doris, Cosmic, Poppy* and *Katy* at the next and last meeting in September.

Wednesday 30 September 2009

Today is the last research group and everyone present had been with the group for five years. Our membership at the end has included *Jonny, Rose, Boris, Doris, Cosmic, Calvin, Poppy, Jenny, Katy* and Heather C – the intrepid 10! Heather C said she could not thank members enough for their huge commitment over these years. A bit of a feast had been provided, including favourites such as a very large chocolate cake, carrot cakes, donuts, and grapes and raspberries for *Cosmic* of course! Those in attendance were also given therapeutic earnings/permitted work payment to say that extra thank you for all they have done. Heather C said she would like to continue to circulate drafts of the chapters being worked on. Currently it is the discussion chapter, and she asked who would like to continue to receive information. Everyone said they would like to continue to receive, read and comment on emerging chapters.

Last month we spent some time asking those present to reflect on what it has meant to be part of the research group. It was agreed to continue this process at the group today.

Jonny, who had given feedback last month, said she wanted to say it had been fun, especially all the talks and conferences. Heather C said that these will continue and, in fact, they could increase.

Boris: It's been a learning curve. It's about believing in yourself and having other people believe in you. It's not just a learning curve about the research project, it's about how we've all changed and grown.

Katy: I enjoyed every minute of it. It was about being understood and helping us to understand each other. I also felt it helped me to remember my BA and academic work. It helped me to think, but it has also helped me to stop dwelling on bad things. I'm going to start a project, 'Five Years at The Haven', starting at the beginning with my experiences and showing how far I have come. I want to interview other people at the project who have been here five years too and I want to keep my brain working.

Doris: If all the clients here were still stuck where they were five years ago, how awful would that be. It's not rocket science – KISS – keep it simple stupid! What it's done for me personally, it's got me into reading more academic literature. That can be quite a struggle when your head's like a washing machine, quite a test.

Cosmic: It was a very productive time. I felt my opinions were really appreciated and that it was a very good project to have been part of, and to have been heard. It was all about self-worth. We could turn it all into a film. George Clooney could play Alan and Meryl Streep could play Heather!

As agreed at earlier meetings, we will now resume the SEGs every six months. A date was fixed for the next one. This will be advertised, run with the same questions, transcribed and distributed, just like it used to be. We will try to get some new people there.

Jonny said, once Heather C has a bit of space in her head for more research, she would still like to see the twin study go ahead at The Haven.

Bye for now and see you later...

Appendix III SEG (Service Evaluation Group) Questions

Question 1: Can you say something about the kinds of responses you have received at The Haven when you have been feeling vulnerable or in crisis?

Question 2: What has been your experience of some of the groups, activities, one-to-ones and other therapies at The Haven?

Question 3: How do you feel The Haven helps you personally?

Question 4: Are you learning new skills which are helping you to understand yourself better?

Question 5: Could you say something about the kinds of coping strategies you have used and whether these have changed?

Question 6: Since coming to The Haven do you feel you spend less time disliking yourself?

Question 7: In what ways, if any, do you feel you have changed as a person since attending The Haven?

Question 8: Is recovery frightening?

Question 8: Can you say something about hopes, dreams and goals for the future, and whether your vision of these have changed since coming to The Haven?

Question 10: What else do you feel The Haven could do to support your recovery?

Appendix IV Client Focus Group Questions

Question 1: Do you feel The Haven helps you personally? If yes how? If no, what would you like The Haven to do for you?

Question 2: Can you say something about the kinds of responses you have received from The Haven when you have been feeling vulnerable or in crisis?

Question 3: What has been your experience of some of the groups, activities and one-to-ones and other therapies at The Haven that you have participated in?

Question 4: Could you say something about The Haven as a community and what this means to you?

Question 5: Are you learning any new skills at The Haven? If so, what do you gain from these new skills?

Question 6: Could you say something about the kinds of coping strategies you have used before coming to The Haven and whether these have changed?

Question 7: Since coming to The Haven do you feel you spend less time disliking yourself?

Question 8: In what ways, if any, do you feel you have changed as a person since attending The Haven?

Question 9: How would you define recovery?

Question 10: Do you think recovery is frightening?

Question 11: Can you say something about hopes, dreams and goals for the future, and whether your vision of these have changed since coming to The Haven?

Question 12: What else do you feel The Haven could do to support you in recovery?

Question 13: Have you got anything more to add?

Appendix V Client Interview Questionnaire

Introduction: Interviewer to introduce themselves and ask the interviewee if they would like to receive a copy of the final results. Assure of confidentiality and explain that the interviewee is free to stop the interview at any point or decline to answer any particular questions. Check that the interviewee is happy to have the interview taped and ask permission to additionally take notes during the interview.

INTERVIEW QUESTIONNAIRE

Gender:	Male ☐		Female ☐
Ethnic origin:			
Age:			
Age range:	18–20 ☐		35–44 ☐
	21–24 ☐		45–54 ☐
	25–34 ☐		55–65 ☐
Marital status:	Single	☐	
	Married/living as	☐	
	Divorced/separated	☐	
	Widowed	☐	
	Other	☐	
Living with:	Alone	☐	
	Partner	☐	
	Partner + children	☐	
	Single parent	☐	
	Parent	☐	
	Others/shared	☐	
Housing:	Own house/flat	☐	

	Rented house/flat	☐	
	Supported accommodation	☐	
	Hospital	☐	
Time at The Haven:	Years _____	Months _____	
Haven services used:	Day services	☐	
	Crisis line	☐	
	Safe centre	☐	
	Crisis/respite bed	☐	

Question 1: Do you feel The Haven helps you personally? If yes how? If no, what would you like The Haven to do for you?

Question 2: How does The Haven compare with other services you have used?

Question 3: Can you say something about the kinds of responses you have received from The Haven when you have been feeling vulnerable and in crisis?

Question 4: What has been your experience of some of the groups, activities and one-to-ones and other therapies at The Haven that you have participated in?

Question 5: Could you say something about The Haven as a community and what this means to you?

Question 6: Do the clients at The Haven interact with and support each other? If yes, how does this work for you?

Question 7: Are you learning any new skills at The Haven? If so, what do you gain from these new skills?

Question 8: Could you say something about the kinds of coping strategies you have used before coming to The Haven and whether these have changed?

Question 9: Since coming to The Haven do you feel you spend less time disliking yourself?

Question 10: In what ways, if any, do you feel you have changed as a person since attending The Haven?

Question 11: How would you define recovery?

Question 12: Do you think recovery is frightening?

Question 13: Can you say something about hopes, dreams and goals for the future, and whether you vision of these have changed since coming to The Haven?

Question 14: What else do you feel The Haven could do to support you in recovery?

Question 15: Have you got anything more to add?

Appendix VI Carer Focus Group Questions

Question 1: Do you think the term 'carer' is appropriate? If not, do you feel another term would be better?

Question 2: Do you feel The Haven has helped the person you support? If yes, how? If no, what would you like The Haven to do for them?

Question 3: Do you feel The Haven involves you in the care offered to the person you support. If yes, how? If no, what would you like The Haven to do to improve this?

Question 4: Research shows that carers often experience difficulties in caring. Do you think this statement is correct and in which way do you think the role affects carers?

Question 5: Are there ways in which you feel you could be supported by The Haven in your role?

Question 6: Do you feel that the person you support has changed since attending The Haven?

Question 7: Do you have hope about the future in relation to the person you support?

Question 8: How would you define recovery?

Question 9: How would you know that the person you are supporting is making progress in their recovery?

Question 10: What else do you feel The Haven could do to help you and the person you support in their recovery?

Question 11: Have you got anything more to add?

Appendix VIII Findings from Client Questions

Do you feel The Haven helps you personally? If yes, how? If no, what would you like The Haven to do for you?

Eight of the 60 clients gave no response to this question.

Fifty clients responded positively and gave a range of ways in which The Haven helps them personally, many stating more than one way.

14 = It is the 24/7 accessibility of The Haven and the fact that there is always someone there who will give me a quick response

Abigail: Its all-round 24-hour support is something that I've really found helpful, knowing that there's someone there; it gives you a sort of safety net.

Jenny: I can come in at any time, or pick up the phone, there's always someone on the other side of the phone.

May: In the hour of need I think, 'The Haven is there'.

11 = It is the caring nature of The Haven that helps me

Ben: I have been met with universal kindness and support.

Gemma: The calmness, softness of the staff they make you feel…they make you a cup of tea or coffee and they listen, they listen. They let you talk, they let you speak, they let you cry and they hand you tissues. You know I never…care and genuine care. Absolutely wonderful!

Phoenix: The Haven provides like a huge big hug.

Norris: It's the sort of place you can get a hug or give one.

Chloe: I don't do hugs, but I do now.

9 = It is acceptance and not being judged at The Haven that helps me

Leska: Being accepted for what I am, with no questions asked. It addresses my own issues and doesn't compare me to everybody else.

Donald: I can be myself without being judged.

Boris: Nobody's going to condemn you, you see the cuts on anyone; they're not going to condemn you.

Katy: In the past two and a quarter years The Haven has supported me, has been non-judgemental and has always been there for me, night or day.

9 = The Haven is somewhere where I am able to express emotions
and be honest

Harry: At The Haven I have permission to show emotion.

Cosmic: It's the only place I've found where I'm taken seriously as somebody with emotional problems.

Luckie: I can be me and express my emotions.

Rose: I find it difficult to show emotion and at The Haven I have permission to show emotion.

8 = The Haven has helped my confidence and self-esteem

Elise: It's been the backbone to make life changes that I've needed to make for a long time.

Alexis: It's reduced the obsessional behaviour and encouraged me to mix with others and it has really boosted my self-esteem.

Ross: It gives me support, boosts confidence and gives me something to focus on. The Haven, for me, it's like having an extra backbone.

Charles: Crisis staff will always try to boost your confidence in some way, they will pull out all the stops to make you try to realize that, you know, your life isn't over and it's not the end of the world.

7 = It is the sense of safety at The Haven that helps me

Harry: The Haven is my safe place.

Igor: It's a safe place. It helps you to be safe.

Katy: Sometimes just what I need at night time is to come in and know I'm safe and it stops me from doing anything at the moment.

Roosle: I'm new to The Haven so I'm just learning what it can do right now. I'm using it as a safe place from myself, because I'm in a very dangerous and unsafe state, and it's a place where I can go where I know I won't come to any harm.

5 = The Haven keeps me stable and able to cope

Rose: It helps me to cope with ups and downs and gets me stabilized when I'm really losing it.

Daniel: It keeps me on an even keel and calms me down.

5 = The Haven helps me to socialize

Alexis: I'm getting out and doing things and meeting people and learning new things; before it was just vegetating at home.

Karen: If I didn't have The Haven to come to I'd be locked in my house most of the time.

Natasha: It gives me a reason to get up to something in the mornings. It helps me to get used to people in a sort of gentle way, you know, sort of like socially.

4 = The Haven has enabled me to trust

Christine: The Haven has taught me to trust again and respect other people. It's through this place I've learnt that I don't have to hide my problems; I don't have to hide behind a smile anymore. I can come in and I can cry and I can be me for once.

Boris: It helps me trust other people and also helps me trust myself more and help myself more.

Anne: I don't have to pretend to be somebody else in front of people who come here because everybody accepts each other, whichever way we come in, happy, sad. I trust everybody here.

3 = The Haven helps me because it is like a family

Pablo: The Haven provides for me a replacement role of my parental home.

Poppy: I'm now learning to use The Haven to help myself and it's like an extended family that I haven't got really.

Ben: It feels that you are a replacement Mum and Dad that I never had.

3 = The Haven helps me by offering practical support

Charles: They helped me when I first came, with getting DLA (disability living allowance) and helping me to secure a flat so that I could be independent.

Jasmine: I've got in a lot of debts and the staff here help me with the paperwork, for which I'm very grateful.

2 = The Haven helps because it has kept me out of hospital

Chloe: I've found The Haven's helped me, I haven't been in (psychiatric hospital) since I've been registered with you, and I haven't been 136'd either.

May: If it wasn't for The Haven I know I would be self-harming. I would also be in hospital now if it wasn't for coming here.

Two clients responded negatively

Kim: Sometimes I don't feel like I'm being taken seriously. Sometimes it feels like it's my paranoia.

Stony: There's people who are ill vying for attention. I feel the one who shouts the loudest gets heard.

How does The Haven compare with other services you have used?

This question was only asked to the twenty clients who were individually interviewed. All responded to the question and 19 responded by making a favourable comparison, most stating more than one point.

10 = The Haven is friendly, caring, welcoming, human and non-judgemental

Doris: It basically knocks them all into a cocked hat…more friendly, relaxed, supportive, and they are quite happy for you to wander off. Whereas, at (another service), you have to sit there for the duration, which is a shame because, at the end of the day, you just turn out being disruptive because you end up annoying other people who want to get on and you don't.

Rose: There's no comparison. The Haven's way and above any of the hospital services I've used and, I'm glad to say I don't have to use inpatient facilities anymore. It's much more personal, and it's complete which helps the whole of you.

Sheila: It's a lot friendlier. It's a lot more caring and it's also trusting. It trusts me a lot more than other services, and you don't get talked down to and treated as though you are some kind of idiot.

Elise: It has a considerate and empathic approach to a situation and it attempts to understand the individual. It has a holistic approach to people's well-being and recovery.

Fred: They treat you like a human being for one and they get to know you as a person and keep up to date with your everyday life really. They are always welcoming.

Carl: They've had to achieve 120 per cent, which no-one on this planet can do, but they're brilliant. They don't judge you and there's no bad feelings.

Brunhilda: It's ten thousand times better than any service I've ever used. In statutory services one definitely felt judged by people. Also, one of the most important things is the humanness of the staff and other clients, there's a kind of warmth and compassion plus The Haven understands the condition of borderline personality disorder.

3 = The Haven is a 24/7 service

Leska: The Haven gives you support 24/7 and you're always reassured that they are there and that you will be able to talk to someone and they care. They address your problems before they get to bad crisis point.

Poppy: It's 24 hours, there's always somebody to contact, whereas with other services they may be open during the day. The groups are much better, and some of the groups focus on specific problems that you have, and it's the only place that's got respite beds.

3 = The Haven is a community

Meg: It compares highly. In fact it's number one. The two main things that stand out is allowing you to become a member of a community, and most organizations I've been to have always tried to reach a discharge date, which sometimes puts a lot of pressure.

Jenny: The community here is so supportive, there's always somebody to talk to and something to do, so you're not sitting and dwelling on how you're feeling. Whereas at (hospital) and other hospitals I've been to, you do.

3 = The Haven is recovery oriented

Pablo: The Haven is consistent, it's been progressive and forward thinking, which is not a stale thing, it's not just something you go back to; it's something you go forward with. Anyone who tries to hold you back, they'll either be back at the (hospital), or back in the situation they were before. If you hang on to The Haven you go forward.

3 = The Haven gives us a voice and choices

Ian: It's a lot better because I feel I have choices. I don't feel like I'm being forced to do things and I come here of my own choice.

Boris: The Haven is completely different to any other service I have ever used. In every other service you don't actually have an opinion or your voice isn't heard. At The Haven your voice is heard and your opinions taken into consideration, and everyone is treated individually here and you're not a number anymore here, you're your own person.

1 = The Haven keeps me out of hospital

Curtis: Before The Haven I tended to be in and out of hospital and that wasn't a very positive experience for any of the time that I was in and out. Hospital is not the ideal place even when I'm not particularly well. The Haven kept me out of hospital, so I have nothing but praise.

One client did not make a favourable comparison

Stony: It's the staff that I have found more helpful than the clients; it's vying for attention again.

Can you say something about the kinds of responses you have received from The Haven when you have been feeling vulnerable or in crisis?

Of the 60 clients who were asked this question, 52 responded and eight did not. Of the 52 clients who answered this question, 50 had positive responses and two did not. Among the 50 who responded positively, nine also made negative comments or suggestions for improvement.

The 50 clients who responded positively gave a range of ways in which The Haven responds to them when they have been feeling vulnerable or in crisis, many stating more than one way.

26 = The Haven has met my needs when I have been feeling vulnerable or in crisis

Katy: They've done exactly what I've needed when I've needed it.

Rose: I've always found the telephone responses very good when I'm in a crisis, they can usually talk me down.

Abigail: I had someone talk me through hyperventilation over the telephone and then talk me back to breathing properly.

Boris: The staff have been really fantastic, whether I've been in day or at night, and all the team have supported me and been there and talked to me if I needed it, or just given me space.

Elise: They've been very responsive. I haven't been pampered when I've been feeling low and vulnerable, or smothered in that sense, but actually people have helped me sit and think things through rationally.

Jasmine: When in crisis the staff go out of their way to see you as soon as they can and I find that really helpful and they help calm you down.

Ross: Good practical advice that puts things into perspective.

Luckie: I was understood and what they said would happen did happen.

19 = The Haven has given me a fast response/is always there when I have been feeling vulnerable or in crisis

Sheila: I've come into the crisis centre someone's always been there immediately. Nobody seems to fob you off onto somebody else.

Ian: There's always been someone to talk to and help me see things differently.

Meg: I've always had immediate response when I've contacted The Haven, every time I've been in crisis, or phoned or texted, I have had a first class response from all members of staff.

Sally: Everybody's been so supportive, there's always somebody there for you.

Abigail: Early intervention, and in my case I was lucky and I had a weekend bed that I wasn't expecting, which was very beneficial.

Katy: They have always been there, day or night, and I can rely on them to support when I need it in crisis.

Tiffany: They do respond to your phone calls and texts quickly to make sure that you don't go down even further. They have always got a friendly smiley face or a nice smiley voice at the end of the phone.

10 = The Haven has responded by getting me into the safe centre or a bed when I have been feeling vulnerable or in crisis

Jenny: I've been in places where I've been feeling very vulnerable, a very bad situation, in crisis, and The Haven will always help me get in here, even if it's by taxi.

Eustace: You can stay overnight for a while under this fantastic roof. I feel everyone around me hated me, until I came here. There's always a smile and a kind word.

Fred: They say come in straight away, they've even booked me a taxi, it doesn't matter how I am, how I'm feeling or what I'm behaving like they still say come in.

Alexis: I've found it very helpful just to come in for a couple of hours and to be amongst people.

Rose: I've always had a good response, I find the calls very helpful and I've even had an admission once in crisis, very quickly arranged.

8 = The Haven has responded in a caring and kind way when I have been feeling vulnerable or in crisis

Doris: It's been excellent, a kind ear, a cuddle, cup of tea, respite when I need it.

Sally: When I have been really down I have been taken into a room and they have made me a cup of coffee and they wouldn't let me out of the door until I have got myself together.

Cosmic: I couldn't wish for more help, more care.

Phoenix: They always look pleased to see you coming through the door.

Fred: I've phoned when I've been in crisis and I've always been welcomed no matter what my mood or what's going through my head.

7 = The Haven has saved my life/saved me from a hospital admission when I have been feeling vulnerable or in crisis

Masie: Four weeks ago I would have ended up in hospital under Section 3 but, because there was intervention, it helped.

Emily: In the past The Haven have sent ambulances which have saved my life.

Crystal: I've had support and kindness, especially all the telephone calls that are regular. If it hadn't been for that I probably wouldn't be here now.

Katy: If it wasn't for The Haven I would have been sectioned, they're there 24/7 and understand.

5 = The Haven has kept me safe or made me feel safe when I have been feeling vulnerable or in crisis

Pablo: You're always acknowledged. It creates security.

Harry: The Haven's my safe space when I get really panicky and, instead of running off and ending in the middle of nowhere, I'm more likely to come here now which actually helps my family a lot because they are not so stressed because they know I am somewhere safe.

Leska: When I've been feeling vulnerable I've always had someone come to talk to me, been reassured that I am safe, and that there are people here to support me and I'm not alone.

4 = The Haven has provided consistency when I have been feeling vulnerable or in crisis

Calvin: There's been concrete, solid support and consistency.

Cosmic: The services here must be fantastic because I haven't been in crisis for ages and ages. It's all about continuity.

May: I think that the way things are handed-over, when you are in crisis you don't have to tell your story all over again from the beginning, because the people you speak to on the phone, or in a one-to-one, know enough about your symptoms and situation and that makes it much easier.

Eleven of the 50 clients also highlighted some occasions when they were not responded to adequately or made suggestions for improvement, and some answered in more than one way.

4 = The Haven did not respond quickly enough or missed calls when I have been feeling vulnerable or in crisis

Christine: Well the only negative experience I've ever had which was a support call that was overlooked, and I was in crisis at the time, but you know, everyone makes mistakes.

Chloe: Down at the old building it seemed to me that the telephone was more important than me because I'd be sitting with somebody in a one-to-one and the minute the phone went they'd be off answering it. I can't compare it because I haven't been here in the new building yet.

Jonny: If there was somebody designated for the phone, you know that the person is designated and they will have to answer it, then you can respond better.

Abigail: I think the staff sometimes cut themselves into lots of little pieces. I actually phoned in the early morning and my brain was telling me to do one thing and I thought I'll phone up and speak to somebody, and, unfortunately, the staff were probably busy with somebody else and it was too late when they did ring me, the situation had happened.

2 = I find it hard to pick up the phone and ask for help when I am feeling vulnerable or in crisis

Sally: Sometimes you can see that staff are all busy, but you're too scared though, and you go home feeling worse, but it's too late. Then it's hard to pick up the phone.

Rose: Sometimes it is hard to pick up the phone so it is better that someone is phoning you.

2 = The Haven has not been caring when I have been feeling vulnerable or in crisis

Harry: I've only had one negative experience, my first response when I got at the door was, 'What time are you going home?'

Leska: Sometimes being let through the front door and nobody actually coming to speak to you for about an hour.

2 = The Haven did not meet my needs when I was feeling vulnerable or in crisis

Boris: Most of the time positive, there are occasions when I talk to staff and I feel they don't actually hear what the problem is.

Gemma: I phoned during the night; I was really desperate and wanted to speak to (staff member). I was told she was busy on the other phone. She didn't offer anything else and I said I'll phone back later and she said okay and put the phone down. She didn't ask how I was. No support, nothing, she just fobbed me off.

1 = The Haven has not been consistent when I have been feeling vulnerable or in crisis

Ben: I've felt a little bit lost because I've been speaking to new members of staff who don't know me and that's made me feel more vulnerable.

Two clients answered only negatively

Kim: I feel I am not always taken seriously.

Norris: I texted in at 2.30pm in the afternoon and got a reply at 5.30pm in the evening.

> What has been your experience of some of the groups, activities and one-to-ones and other therapies at The Haven that you have participated in?

Of the 60 clients who were asked this question, 52 answered and eight did not. All 52 responded positively, but seven of these also commented negatively, or with comments or suggestions. Their comments are included within each category of activity. Most clients cited a number of activities at The Haven.

One-to-ones
18 = Responded positively about one-to-one work

Doris: They make you feel that, for half an hour, you are the sole focus of their attention. You're not just a number and you've got these issues and they are going to sit there and listen to you. Even if it goes over, they are not clock-watching. There's no 'I'm going to get my lunch now.' You are important.

Curtis: The one-to-ones I have, like focused one-to-ones; I find really useful and also like sort of grounding yourself.

Abigail: They are quite inspirational and they make you come away and think. You might not always agree with what's been said at the time, but I have time to reflect and I think that's one of the benefits of having one-to-ones.

Boris: I like my one-to-ones because I have a chance to be me, I can let my barriers down, I can say how I am really feeling, I can vent myself when I am angry, and I can talk through every emotion that I am feeling and the troubles I am struggling with at the time.

Lara: I am really grateful for the one-to-ones so I can let it all out, and the staff that help me I can't give them enough credit because they really do help put you at ease.

Crystal: I find the one-to-ones very useful, although it can bring up the past and it's extremely painful, but is helping in the long-term.

Charles: I've been using the one-to-ones; it's a way forward for me if I'm feeling angry I vent my anger.

Brunhilda: I've felt the focused one-to-ones very helpful because you can get to grips with something, a particular something, and there's continuity.

Poppy: The one-to-ones are extremely important.

Groups

18 = Responded

15 = Responded positively about the group program in general

Brunhilda: There's such a nice wide variety of groups and activities and it feels as if there is something for everyone.

Natasha: It's just that there's something to do all the time. They encourage you to do things but there's no pressure.

Chloe: The comparison that springs to mind is with the groups that are run here, with the groups run in typical institutions and hospital settings that is, and it's just worlds apart and you don't feel like you're in a group. Well personally I don't feel I'm in a group just to pass the time, there's loads more to it than that. It's about social interaction, it's about learning, it's about all sorts of things, and you feel, you know, you do feel good afterwards.

Pablo: They have been educational and fun.

Rose: I'm talking more, getting more involved with groups and I've found this is helping me feel more part of the community.

Boris: What I like is when there isn't a member of staff available to run the group we are asked if we would like to do it.

Cosmic: The groups are excellent, the way you can just turn up for a group, I find that very supportive. I know that's in my diary, I like the group, and I turn up.

Phoenix: This is the first time in life I've felt safe in a group.

Katy: I think a lot of effort has gone into the groups and I think they are very beneficial to everybody.

3 = Responded negatively or with comments or suggestions about groups

Curtis: Groups stress me out.

Rose: I find groups overwhelming.

Christine: I find it very difficult to start in joining groups that have already been established for a while, so I might need some encouragement or a size 9 behind me to help me join in.

DBT (dialectical behaviour therapy skills group)

13 = Responded
10 = Responded positively

Pablo: I'm learning to tolerate people; I'm not so judgemental of people. I know that's a DBT skill.

Harry: DBT has been teaching us mindfulness exercises, which I have got to say have helped me enormously, because I used to suffer from really bad road rage and generally I can control it now.

Lara: I attend DBT because I can see how much enjoyment people get out of it. I think it's helped me tremendously. I used to go off the handle at anything, now I stop to think of a different way of coping with it and a different way of speaking to people and it's much more effective than just lashing out.

Natasha: I find DBT's been very helpful especially with negative thoughts and coping skills, mindfulness.

Charles: Mindfulness, to my knowledge, is about being mindful of others and say, for instance, someone is throwing a temper tantrum and acting aggressively, you have to think to yourself there's a reason. How would I feel if I was doing that, because I have thrown temper tantrums here? What I'm trying to say is the next time I throw a temper tantrum I should really and truly be thinking about how I am affecting other people.

Brunhilda: DBT I have found very interesting and helpful. It's a particularly difficult module at the moment that we are doing, called distress tolerance, and I think it's quite good that I've noticed that one or two members of staff know a little bit about it as well and that's helpful because I can discuss it in a one-to-one. But for other clients it could be quite helpful as well because I'm sure more people would be in DBT if it were possible, so some staff knowing about it passes on the benefits.

3 = Responded negatively or with comments or suggestions

Stony: I found that didn't help me because I looked too much in my past.

Doris: I started DBT; I didn't click with the group. There were some members of the group that seemed to consider it their group and they bullied and took over the place, so I wasn't prepared for it. I wasn't going to have that, and when I feel like doing DBT again it won't be when they are in the group.

Harry: It's the lack of reminders because when you do DBT anywhere else you have a one-to-one session during the week to help to remind you of your skills and you are supposed to be practicing and obviously here we haven't got that.

Reflexology
13 = Responded positively

Emily: I hate being touched and I actually let a member of staff do my feet.

Lucy: Reflexology I have also had and that's helped me to chill out, and unwind, it was nice.

Karen: Reflexology is brilliant, I never felt so calm.

Rose: Reflexology is good; I nearly fell asleep three times.

Cosmic: Reflexology, that was great, that was good; she's a brilliant listener too.

Carl: I've had reflexology and that's very good, it calms you down, makes you feel good, sometimes it helps with answers which has been related to the problem, to yourself, to your body, and then it can be washed away, or that's what I found.

Friendship groups

12 = Responded
11 = Responded positively

Chloe: I think the friendship groups are the best groups. I think people tend to interact, peer-support. I haven't laughed as much in years at the last friendship group I came to here. It was just hilarious.

Doris: Friendship group I love, especially now it's more structured, like we're doing bingo and having a bit more of a laugh.

Sally: I find friendship group has helped, because if I'm down they always cheer you up.

Wilf: Friendship groups, even sitting about talking, you can see by some people that they have been as low as you have, we've all been down, right to that bottom, hell really isn't it, and that I think helps you to talk to people, open up, because they've been through the same sort of pain.

May: Friendship groups make me feel part of a family.

1 = Responded negatively or with comments or suggestions

Stony: I found friendship group not that helpful because, while I was there people were talking about their illnesses and competing over their illnesses, and I didn't find that very helpful at all.

Transitional recovery group
11 = Responded
10 = Responded positively

Doris: I love transitional recovery, I absolutely love it. I think it's the group I get the absolute most out of, and I know that quite a lot of people here feel the same. It's a very empowering group, it's a group that gives you a chance to move on. It helps give you the tools to move on.

Stony: That's why I've started coming back, because there's methods for helping people who do want to move on.

Boris: It helps build confidence and helps you build new friendships and support one another, and it's really productive and really positive. Last week was really good hearing people's goals and looking at what stopped us achieving them.

Bling: It was a great opportunity for us to go on that outward pursuits, outward bounds for the day.

Fred: Transitional Recovery, I'm finding that really helpful, it's helping me find college courses and helping the route I actually wanted to go down, whereas I couldn't really pin the route I wanted to be on. Now I know how to get to that route, finding those bridges to cross. So I'm on the right path now which makes so much difference in my life. I know it's achievable now.

1 = Responded negatively or with comments or suggestions

Brunhilda: I personally haven't been much to it, and I think that's because I'd quite like there to be some connection to one-to-ones because I actually don't feel very comfortable to be in that group. I think it might be something to do with being older and perhaps, I've done courses, you know careers, that kind of thing doesn't seem quite appropriate for me, so I don't know. I'm just quite confused about it.

Creative writing group
11 = Responded positively

Gemma: The writers' group, writing things down, I use that as a coping strategy.

Jonny: Writing group, there is a lot of honesty. It's been like that more or less from the beginning. But I've been surprised by what I've written.

Anne: I am finding creative writing extremely helpful, it's helping me to get a lot of my emotions out on to paper and being able to share them with other people as well has always been hard for me, but I've started to read out my work.

Doris: Writing group gets things out of my head.

Natasha: Creative Writing, a good skill to have. I may write a book one day!

Donald: It has definitely given me a chance to say what I feel, and write down my feelings, which has been really, really helpful, and just listening to what other people have written, as well, it can be really insightful.

Arts and crafts group
9 = Responded positively

Harry: The art group, it gives you time away from your problems, it helps you to focus on something else rather than what's causing you distress.

Phoenix: Arts and crafts is brilliant.

Daniel: I'm not good at art but I attend. You can wander in and out if you like.

Norris: We've done things like clay model making. I have gone home and got some clay. Me and my daughter have been doing that. That's like a distraction.

Life skills group
8 = Responded
7 = Responded positively

Alexis: I feel I've really benefited from the life skills group; it's reduced my obsessional behaviour and encouraged me to mix with others and has really boosted my self-esteem. It's been very beneficial dealing with anxiety, positive thinking, how to control panic attacks, confidence building and particularly in dealing with anger.

Cosmic: The life skills is brilliant because it's so varied, and I've learned a lot and it's good to be re-running the course as well, because if there's anything that I've missed, or wasn't paying attention.

Sally: Some of it's hard this week but brilliant.

Brunhilda: I think life skills is pretty good to do it the second time around, it makes more sense, so I like that rolling program.

1 = Responded negatively or with comments or suggestions

Ben: I find the life skills group very threatening, so much so, I haven't been able to sit through a whole one yet.

Gardening group
8 = Responded positively

Sheila: Gardening Group is just good physical exercise which I appreciate and you can have a laugh with other people while you are doing it, and obviously making things look nice.

Abigail: The work that has been done by everybody that goes, and personally I was shown photos of people that I have never seen smile before, which to me is what it's all about.

Crystal: I love gardening. I think it is beautiful to see things grow.

Daniel: Do people feel proud of the gardening group, well the ones that are doing it, yea!

Pampering
8 = Responded positively

Kim: I love the face packs, or my hands being done, I feel like a queen.

Rose: Pampering, you feel so much better you do, you feel like a real person.

Chloe: The only time I'm really touched is when I come here, because I live by myself and don't have a partner. The pampering is a clear example of somebody actually touching you and that makes you feel that you are valuable as a person by being actually touched. Touch is really important.

Harry: I found pampering particularly good because I don't pamper myself and it's nice to feel you're worth something through having that done. I'm starting to learn that I'm not just what I do, I am a person as well and that I have needs.

Counselling
7 = Responded
6 = Responded positively

Rose: The counselling I'm receiving, I have been for quite a while, is just fantastic. I've had ten years of psychotherapy; I've still managed to avoid the issues. With the counselling I think it's the fact that it's here. It makes me feel safer which makes me take more risks than I ever have.

Sally: I find counselling very good and very helpful. It's helped me to talk freely and be able to trust other people.

May: I also have counselling once a week and I feel very safe talking to her, and she says it's my time, it's my space. I talk about what I want, and I'm not pushed to talk about anything I don't want to but I'm encouraged to talk about other things I find difficult.

1 = Responded negatively or with comments or suggestions

Curtis: I did have a few weeks of counselling, but it was at a time when things were very bad, and it was too much.

Other activities
7 = Responded positively

263

Elise: I like helping with Open Days and the neighbours.

Brunhilda: I'm a member of The Haven Hat Society!

Emily: I was quite apprehensive about joining. I wondered what kind of stories and how in-depth we had to go, but it turned out to be very light and very entertaining (Personality+ storytelling session).

Daniel: I've noticed it with the dog that even people that are in stressful situations, when the dog walks in it will spot that and it will come over to them. We want more of the Pat Dog.

Health and fitness group
6 = Responded positively

Fred: Health and fitness I like as well, it's got me going swimming and generally eating better because I feel better about myself.

Ross: Health and fitness, this helps my inner body, eases pain and helps me control my breathing, also gives me a chance to get out and about be it walking or swimming.

Brunhilda: I always feel better after doing it.

Other complementary therapies (head massage, hand reflexology)
6 = Responded positively

Tom: Head massage helps the pain in my head it does.

Crystal: I'm not a very touchy person because I haven't been brought up like that but I found what I had yesterday was really calming and I felt good afterwards.

Substance misuse support group
3 = Responded positively

Emily: Substance misuse group is brilliant and everyone was so honest last week about where they were at, I found it very humbling and overwhelming the honesty in that group.

Nutrition group
2 = Responded positively

Daniel: It's really beneficial, she's really clued up.

Chaplaincy group
2 = Responded positively

Jonny: It's great when we've got the blokes there. It gives a more even balance.

Drumming group
2 = Responded positively

Brunhilda: It's great because you can't think about anything else at all, when you're drumming, it's impossible.

Could you say something about The Haven as a community and what this means to you?

Of the 60 clients in the sample, 15 were not asked this question as it was not included in the earlier service evaluation groups. Of the 45 respondents who were asked this question, five did not respond. Of the 40 who did respond, 38 responded positively, many stating in more than one way.

14 = The Haven community helps me to feel accepted, valued and not judged

Katy: I think it's very important it's a community. I think being non-judgemental against each other is very important, and I think it's very important that it's become a very close community.

Rose: I have a valid point of view. It's very important to me, the fact that it's a community made up of so many different people. There can be underlying things going on, but that's because it's a community. It's no different to the outside world.

Cosmic: The atmosphere and the feeling of the community is just getting better and better and it's reached a peak for me, there's no more cliqueyness and it's really straightened itself out now.

Sally: We're very respectful of one another, the staff as well. We talk to each other as an equal.

Bling: The community aspect is really good, no-one picks on anyone, it's not a place where people pick on each other, there's no piss taking, there's no nasty bullying which you get elsewhere.

Elise: It's nice to have a cosy little environment where everybody gets on with everybody, but that isn't a true reflection of how it is in the real world and it's actually accepting differences and understanding that that's how things are.

Leska: You know you are not going to be judged, people are going to accept you for who you are, what mood you are in.

Tiffany: No-one is putting a label on each other like they do everywhere else.

Emily: I find when you walk into the room, the thing I like about all of them is, everybody has got the same illness, same problems, and this is where The Haven comes into its own, and walking into the room, people talk to you, they don't judge you, nothing like that, so I feel good.

11 = The Haven community can provide mutual support

Meg: Client interaction is vital. We are all prepared to assist each other.

Anne: It's what The Haven is all about; it's being there for each other through good times and bad.

Katy: The support we give each other is absolutely fantastic.

Pablo: There's great interaction between the clients at The Haven and the support is good.

Poppy: I get good support from the other clients.

9 = The Haven community can provide friendship and togetherness

Doris: It's all about human contact. I think a lot of people here realize what it's like to be lonely, we all know what it's like so we all make an extra effort to be friendly, to be nice; to make a cup of tea. Ah bless, I love the community at The Haven. I love all the friends I've made. I love all the people I wouldn't normally have spoken to.

Sally: I'd be lost without The Haven, everyone seems so friendly, all the clients seem so friendly, and make you feel welcome.

Gemma: There's always people around and you can hear them laughing, precious company.

Christine: Having somewhere like this to come takes away part of the loneliness and I've made a lot of good friends.

Donald: A Sunday roast because it was my birthday on Sunday made me feel really good and happy. It was one of the best birthdays I ever had.

7 = The Haven community is about working together

Boris: It's a whole big box of people together that are all striving for the same thing and the community is what you make it, and what you give to it, and how much people are willing to put into it.

Jonny: It's a learning curve for all of us, working as a team, staff and clients.

Jenny: I think The Haven works because it is a community, we all work together, and any problems that do arise we all get together and decide what's going to happen.

Fred: Everyone pulls together; I feel part of it now.

Brunhilda: It's such a great representation of what you would call a community, and I personally have looked for a community for several years and this is really what I think community ought to be, because it's staff and clients all together have created this place.

5 = The Haven community is a very different way of running things

Rose: I haven't seen any NHS mental health people run things like this.

Jenny: I don't think I've ever been any place where there's been people around me that have got mental health problems and there's been such a good strength of community.

Ross: The community meetings are good. It's a chance for the clients to advise on what is required as a community. Having a say is a big step forward in our recovery.

Wilf: It's brilliant that we run it, and we decide what happens. I mean it's not, it's never nice to ban people and things like that, but at certain times we have to be stricter. I think it's important that we do run it and we decide everything, really, don't we?

5 = The Haven community helps me to understand and feel understood

Emily: I isolate and can't mix with people, but I can see people in The Haven, you are the same as me.

Meg: It's the community and having people here who understand you.

Phoenix: Being around other people when you've been socially secluded for so long, in itself, teaches you new skills, to re-learn and re-define.

4 = The Haven community is a way I can help others

Sheila: I enjoy cooking for people, cakes and things.

Lara: I just love helping people. I feel that when I'm helping someone it makes me feel better.

4 = The Haven community is like a family

Boris: It's like one big family together. You support one another through your needs.

Leska: The Haven community, it means a lot to me, it's like having a family all under one roof.

May: It's the family I never had.

Seven clients responded negatively. Of those seven, five had also responded positively, above, and two responded only negatively.

4 = The Haven community makes me feel threatened or that I can't fit in

Sheila: I would like to be able to join in the community more, but I'm not very good at interacting with other people I suppose.

Kim: Sometimes I do feel alone at the groups, I feel there's a lot of cliqueyness and bullying going on. Maybe it's a clash of personality and I feel it should be looked at.

Phoenix: I struggle with this idea of community. Sometimes I feel very, very threatened, and sometimes I feel very safe, sometimes I feel comforted, but there are times I feel threatened and vulnerable.

3 = The Haven community can be about illness rather than recovery

Ian: Sometimes it's unhelpful if people were telling me things that they have done that are not good.

Stony: The Haven as a community isn't that good really, to be honest, because people are, like I said over again, focusing on the actual illness rather than trying to move forward with everything, and everybody's competing on how ill they are rather than trying to be better.

Cosmic: I think alcoholism isn't named for what it is. I think there's too many people that are not using self-management skills and becoming independent. I don't see The Haven as a place to land, it's a place to touch down and spring from.

Are you learning any new skills at The Haven? If so, what do you gain from these new skills?

Of the 60 clients who were asked this question, 12 did not respond. The remaining 48 gave positive responses, many highlighting more than one skill.

11 = I am learning therapeutic skills at The Haven

Harry: I was very fortunate to have DBT here, and we've done mindfulness and I've found that extremely useful, and I try to do it every day now, at least once a day.

Cosmic: Life skills is brilliant, so varied, I've learned a lot.

Lara: I'm learning an awful lot in DBT, mindfulness, thinking before you speak, trying to change your actions and the way you think.

Karen: Life skills group is excellent. I've learned a lot from life skills.

Donald: I'm doing CBT and I find that very helpful. I feel I've come a long way since I came here three months ago and I'm pretty proud.

Poppy: I feel by going to life skills and transitional recovery groups it's given me the confidence to go to college.

9 = I am learning academic skills at The Haven

Doris: My maths is pretty much diabolical and, through the transitional recovery group, I've found that it's not perhaps as diabolical.

Christine: From the Bridges to Education workshop I've learned the new skills of having to go back to college, hopefully in September.

Jenny: Transitional group again, is getting me back into retraining my brain again, getting me like practising English papers and maths papers.

Fred: I'm learning some maths, because I'm useless at maths, and I need it to go on in college.

9 = I am learning to change my negative coping strategies at The Haven

Masie: I've stopped cutting, I haven't done anything for eight months now.

Elise: I think my new skills have fundamentally been to be able to stop and question the reality of the situation and the most logical conclusions, and the most logical assumptions, and to think the whole situation through, rather than jump into the first panic stricken thought that comes into my head and act on it. It's the actual stopping and analysing the situation for what it really is, not what emotionally it's built itself up to be. That's the best skills I've learned.

Ben: I'm learning I don't have to be ill to be loved.

Rose: I used to cut but can have sharp knives in the kitchen now. My negative coping strategies, like opening a bottle of wine, are changing to picking up the telephone and leaving the wine in the fridge.

Katy: I have learned different strategies especially how to control my substance misuse.

Jasmine: I used to self-harm a lot and with help of staff in one-to-ones I've now started to recognize when I'm heading down that path and be able to phone before I actually do something.

Fred: I'm also clean and have stayed clean. That time they booked me the taxi I could have gone back to using without even knowing it was wrong, which I have done in the past, whilst I've been psychotic still. Kind of like instead of popping a pill, I come here.

9 = I have learned to communicate better and trust more at The Haven

Rose: I've learned a lot of new skills from The Haven. I've learned to talk more openly to share how I'm actually feeling, rather than covering it up. I've learned to trust which enables me to talk which is a major breakthrough.

Boris: I've learned to share my feelings more instead of keeping them inside. Before, I was always frightened to express how I felt, if I got locked up, in case I was rejected again.

Anne: I've learned to trust more and it's helped me to be more open.

Luckie: I'm more truthful about myself and who I am. I'm not pretending to be something I'm not.

Ross: I think the new skills I'm learning at The Haven at the moment are interaction and communication.

7 = I have learned skills that are of practical use outside The Haven

Sheila: I am learning to talk a bit more and that helps me outside. Just mundane things like going to the bank, I can actually speak to people behind the counter without just standing there and grunting at them.

Stony: A bit more independence, a student has taken me out on the bus to help me get used to buses.

Leska: One of the biggest new skills I'm learning is how to be a Mum, and I suppose another big skill I'm learning is to try and stand on my own two feet and try to deal with stuff, instead of asking The Haven for so much support, how to be patient, how to interact with someone who can't talk, and to love someone who's so dependent on you, learning to love you could say.

Tiffany: When I'm in a crowd I used to have to walk out, now I find I can stay in a crowd a little bit longer. It's a skill for me to actually get on a bus and a train. Without the tools that The Haven has given us; then I don't think I would have been able to have done it.

7 = I have learned to be able to socialize better at The Haven

Doris: I think one of the paramount skills I've learned since my time at The Haven was how to make a decent cup of tea! I've learned listening, I've learned how to make friends, and it's helped me to realize that I'm not such a pile of shit anymore.

Fred: I'm learning not to isolate so much and to, you know, be around people.

Carl: I'm learning to re-socialize, have fun with other people, joining in and laughs, and general well-being.

6 = I have learned to ask for help when I need it at The Haven

Rose: I am learning to actually ask for help before I act on things.

Sally: I just used to sit in my flat and suffer in silence, but now I'm picking up the phone.

Katy: I can call in from home and I've also been able to ask for help which is really new.

Jasmine: I find since I've been coming here I've been able to sort of open up what I bottle up inside, and that it is okay sometimes to ask for help when you need it.

6 = My self-awareness has increased since coming to The Haven

Kim: I feel more aware of my insecurities.

Harry: I've been learning where a lot of my difficulties have stemmed from which is, hopefully, in the long term, helping me to overcome them.

Charles: I've learned a lot about myself, that I've got problems in certain areas, sort of anger and stuff like that, and you know, alcoholism.

5 = I am learning tolerance and acceptance at The Haven

Pablo: I have more tolerance, I'm less judgemental and more patient.

Abigail: I'm learning to be more tolerant of others because I always expected others to be as I expect myself to be and I am a very harsh person, so I am learning to be more tolerant.

Jonny: You're not chastised for slipping back if you do slip back. I think everybody who comes here learns to be more tolerant.

5 = I am learning how to be more confident at The Haven

Anne: I'm learning to be more confident in what I do, I'm getting a lot more confident also in learning to talk to other clients here, and I can be relaxed enough to be myself.

Fred: I gain confidence and self-esteem.

Cosmic: I've had the confidence to start voluntary work because you had the confidence in me to show me the advert, see, for the job, so there.

Boris: I suppose the dominant skill I'm learning at The Haven is being more confident that I can achieve more than I think I can.

3 = I am learning hope at The Haven

Wilf: Seeing the people who have moved on to college and stuff, you can set yourself a little goal then, can't you. They've done it, so you know, maybe there's a chance.

Milly: I think that transitional recovery group gives you a lot of hope.

2 = I am improving/regaining old skills at The Haven

Ian: I'm learning to use skills, I know, better.

Cosmic: Brushing up on old ones, self-management skills.

One client also responded negatively

Ben: No I'm not. All my one-to-ones are spent with me blubbing and them offering me tissues, but no way I've been taught techniques to help myself.

Could you say something about the kinds of coping strategies you have used before coming to The Haven and whether these have changed?

Of the 60 clients who were asked this question, nine did not respond. The remaining 51 gave answers ranging from a dramatic reduction in the use of negative coping strategies, a reduction, to no change or setbacks.

23 = Since coming to The Haven there has been a dramatic reduction in my use of negative coping strategies

Pablo: My sobriety is unbelievable, my conscience is clear, I wake up clear. I mean the two things in my life that I do now that keep me together is that I eat well and I sleep well.

Anne: Before The Haven existed I was self-harming on a very regular basis, cutting and overdosing, but since coming here it's stopped, they both have.

Doris: They've changed dramatically. I used to be cutting, drinking too much and speeding off in my car and I think I've cut once in the past year.

Rose: I haven't cut for more than two years now, my overdosing has gone down significantly, and my drinking is getting to be more normal.

Sally: I haven't self-harmed for six months now. I normally phone The Haven up. Before I used to run away if I'd got problems, but now I don't, I face up to the problems I've got.

Chloe: My coping strategies are completely different now. I have not self-harmed this year. I channel my feelings and emotions more constructively. I do a lot of sport now.

Elise: Before I came to The Haven I used to overdose on a reasonably regular basis, I used to cut myself when anything went wrong. Basically, it was a whole host of maladaptive coping mechanisms and since coming to

The Haven I have sort of redressed these. A lot of the reason has been because of the ruling about coming in when you have cut, or coming in when you have drunk alcohol. So you have to respect the values of the place. I now don't cut. To me to cut would be such a backward step I don't even want to go there.

Christine: I used two forms of negative strategies before I came here and it's now over seven months since I've done either.

Leska: Before I came to The Haven nearly every other day I was tying things around my neck, overdosing, cutting myself and since coming to The Haven I don't tie anything round my neck, I've had maybe one overdose and I've learned to talk and, when things get really bad, to phone and ask for support instead of acting on impulsive thoughts.

Alexis: I haven't touched alcohol for almost two years. I haven't self-harmed for almost 19/20 months with the help of The Haven's crisis line.

Tiffany: My coping strategies was drinking, taking drugs, overdosing and harming myself, and now I don't do any of those things since coming to The Haven. The staff, they make you feel really guilty about trying to do something like that! The next day you might wake up and think, oh my God, I am so glad I didn't do anything.

Fred: Taking drugs, before in the past, that was all I knew from the age of 13, what I'd learned in order to survive, basically, on the streets. I've come beyond that and my coping strategies are to talk I guess, and phone for help.

Donald: I used to overdose probably once or twice a week and, in the last four or five months, that's stopped completely since I've come here. I never used to think about the consequences, I never used to think about who I was going to hurt, I never used to think there were other ways of dealing with things, and that you could actually talk to someone about things, instead of just doing it, so it's changed my life no end coming here.

13 = Since coming to The Haven there has been a reduction in my use of negative coping strategies

Boris: They have decreased. Here I have broken the cycle of the pattern of behaviour into more constructive ways of dealing with it. Self-harming, or picking up a bottle of wine, I tend more now to put pen to paper and let it out that way.

Abigail: I didn't used to eat properly, but I eat three times a day now. I used to drink as well and one of the reasons why I don't drink in the evenings if I'm feeling really bad is just in case I need to come in here. It makes me think, 'No you can't go in there if…'

Calvin: I can call in here now rather than pick up a drink.

Jenny: I used to self-harm a lot before I came here. Instead of doing that I've managed to pick up the phone. I used to like drink quite a lot as well, and knowing that if I do I can't come in here and speak to somebody, and I'd rather speak to somebody rather than pick up a drink.

10 = Since coming to The Haven there is beginning to be a reduction in my use of negative coping strategies

Kim: Cutting has lightened up a bit because I have used the phone.

Ruth: I smoked a lot of cannabis but managed to give up two weeks ago.

Phoenix: I've used all sorts of negative, self-harming behaviour and it's probably too early for me. But I think the one thing I have noticed is that I'm more inclined to pick up the phone before I start drinking now.

5 = Since coming to The Haven I have not reduced my use of negative coping strategies

Ben: I've hung on to my coping strategies which are distinctly negative because I feel that if I give them up then I'm lost. I've got nothing to replace them with, so I'm not willing to give them up yet.

Natasha: I've started using cannabis again in the evenings, but I haven't been coming here long, well that's a bit of a confession isn't it!

Harry: At the moment my self-harm has got a lot worse. But I'm going through a very difficult period at the moment and the thing I have to realize is that, although I'm getting less judgemental of other people, I'm getting more judgemental with myself. So I'm actually, at the moment, more likely to self-harm but I'm less likely to get myself into a fight with someone else.

Since coming to The Haven do you spend less time disliking yourself?

Of the 60 clients who were asked this question, 12 did not respond. The remaining 48 answered 'yes', expressed tentative improvements, or answered 'no'. Answers have also been categorized in relation to how long respondents have been clients at The Haven.

17 = Who have been at The Haven for two to three years answered 'yes'

Pablo: Yea I have started liking myself more, definitely, and I would squarely put some of that help in The Haven's ball court.

Boris: I think it's more about being comfortable with who I am. I'm content with who I am at this moment in time.

Anne: Yes I do. I used to really hate myself. I feel a lot better with the help from staff and clients. They have really helped me to start to see myself for who I am.

Leska: I know something has changed because I don't feel like a thing anymore. I have more time to try and like myself.

Elise: I now find things to like about myself, and I go out and treat myself to nice clothes because they will make me look nice, and get my nails done.

Bling: Absolutely, definitely, yes!

Fred: I think how far I have come. When I think of that, I think no, I have done really well, and I know now, it's not an excuse, things that happened to me while I was in care and on the street, it wasn't my fault.

Harry: I think I used to dislike myself a lot. I don't actually dislike myself now, although I dislike my behaviour at times, which is a massive difference and I'm actually able to go out and buy new clothes. So being able to spend money on myself has come from being at The Haven and being made to feel worthwhile.

Carl: I feel human again and not an outcast.

Brunhilda: At The Haven you get so much positive feedback and just logically, if quite a lot of people think that you are a decent human being, logically you must be. Eventually, yes, you get re-programmed, it definitely does filter through.

5 = Who have been at The Haven for one to two years answered 'yes'

Tiffany: The staff make you feel special in your own way. I am beginning to believe in myself a little bit more than I have ever done in my life.

Natasha: I think I do like myself a bit more than I did.

3 = Who have been at The Haven for less than one year answered 'yes'

Chloe: There are things about myself that I do like. There are qualities and parts of my character that I think are as valuable and specific to me. So I value myself, so yes I do spend less time disliking myself.

Milly: Yes I'm feeling more able to look at communicating with people differently, and getting better results, so I suppose it's improved my self-esteem.

4 = Who have been at The Haven for two to three years expressed tentative improvements

Jonny: There's less time to think about it, but it's very deep rooted, the very core.

Katy: I still have a problem, I feel very worthless, but when I'm on the premises I like myself, coming helps me to like myself.

Rose: I spend less time disliking myself, I get out more, don't feel quite so useless.

2 = Who have been at The Haven for one to two years expressed tentative improvements

Lara: I like myself here but I don't like myself at home. I still can't look in the mirror.

5 = Who have been at The Haven for less than one year expressed tentative improvements

Ian: I dislike less, I think so.

Christine: I don't dislike myself less just I spend less time thinking about it.

Karen: Not all of the time, but hopefully as time goes by I will start liking myself.

4 = Who have been at The Haven for two to three years answered 'no'

Sally: I still dislike myself. I don't know if it will ever change, it's always as far as I can remember for such a long time ago, that's just how I feel about myself.

Jasmine: No I still hate myself but my feelings here have changed, I'm not 136'd so often now, the police station used to be my second home.

2 = Who have been at The Haven for one to two years answered 'no'

Charles: I'd like to think I like myself more, loud and brash, but behind closed doors I'm pretty depressed.

6 = Who have been at The Haven for less than one year answered 'no'

Kim: I hate myself, my self-esteem is so low.

Masie: I feel I spend more time disliking myself because I see hordes of people out there, in here, that are able to cope with life and I don't feel worthy.

Ruth: I still hate myself.

Crystal: No I haven't learned to like myself, there's a long way to go.

In what ways, if any, do you feel you have changed as a person since attending The Haven?

Of the 60 clients who were asked this question, 11 did not respond. Of the remaining 49, 46 answered positively and many responded in a variety of ways, some highlighting more than one change.

22 = Since The Haven I have changed as a person by becoming more confident

Ian: More confident and more able to talk to people, slightly more outgoing I suppose, and I laugh a lot more than I did.

Rose: I now speak up for myself. I have a lot more confidence in the community.

Boris: I am stronger in my beliefs and I fight for what I think is correct.

Harry: My confidence has risen enormously. A year and a half ago I was never leaving the house. I like the fact that when I do the personality disorder awareness training all the professionals there, they're actually looking up to me, and that's a big thing because I've always had very low self esteem.

Cosmic: I think I've gone down from PD platinum to PD bronze! The idea is to work your way down isn't it? I've found that, since being in a group situation, it means it jars your confidence to leave this room and go and join other groups.

Elise: Fundamentally, it's given me the confidence to go and be my own person and to leave the relationship that was holding me back as a person, and that's been because I know I've got the support here that

I can now go and stand on my own two feet. I've got a lot more self-respect, my self-esteem's definitely improved, but it's basically self-respect.

Jasmine: I never used to like going on public transport or getting in a car because of panic attacks, but since I've been here I've been able to get on trains and on the bus, and getting on the taxi run.

Jenny: My confidence as well has gone up a lot. It's not that I'm a diagnosis. I understand a lot more about it and I've got support from here, so I know my rights, and I know what to say really.

Tiffany: Staff and clients build you up and make you feel very confident about yourself.

Daniel: Since I've been coming here I've actually gone to several conferences and had enough courage to speak as one of the guests.

16 = Since attending The Haven I have changed as a person by learning things about myself

Doris: I've learned a lot about myself. I rediscovered the fact that I am good, I am not as bad as I think I am.

Chloe: I actually feel that my behaviour has changed. It's become, in nursing jargon, more appropriate, it's less extreme the majority of the time.

Harry: I am a lot more insightful into my condition. I pick up on things earlier so I can sort of try to change, avert a crisis before it happens.

Max: I'd like to think I'm not quite as impulsive as I was.

Connar: Trying to help other people to distract from your own personal issues and problems and facing up to your own demons, by distracting from my personal issues what I was doing was making them worse, so that's what I've learnt from that.

Katy: I've changed in lots of different ways and I've learned that the voices I hear are actually in my head.

Poppy: I don't get stroppy anymore and walk out in a huff. Although the depression has been really awful and painful at times, I think I've learned more about it and I realize, by talking to a lot of other people, not just at The Haven, that there's a lot of depression around, and I think it's made me more caring and sincere towards other people's problems.

Daniel: I don't boss people about, I'm not as aggressive. I used to be a big bully.

12 = Since attending The Haven I have changed as a person by becoming more sociable and better at communicating

Ross: I'm far less arrogant and pretentious and self-centred and I try to think of others.

Cosmic: I feel more secure. I used to feel like a freak. Why am I so different from the neighbours? But this is a whole club full of them and I keep in mind that I'm not alone.

Carl: I can now have a conversation and make a conversation.

Diana: I'm re-engaging with clients and staff, talking a lot more. I used to sit there and say nothing, but now I'm talking.

Daniel: I've come out of my shell.

10 = Since attending The Haven I have changed as a person by becoming more open and trusting

Boris: I'm more honest, I'm more open, I'm more trusting since coming to The Haven, and I've managed to drop my barriers more, a lot more than I ever used to since coming here. I've been able to let more people in.

Norris: When I first came here I couldn't let anyone near me, or in my space, without being completely drunk, this was outside here, and now I can. Most of the time people can hug me and be close to me without, you know, that would have never happened before I started coming here, without me being under the influence.

Poppy: I've opened up quite a lot. I used to hide my feelings because I was told that it was a bad thing to show feelings, it was a sign of weakness.

Brunhilda: I'm more able to demonstrate affection without feeling too vulnerable.

9 = Since attending The Haven I have changed as a person because I am beginning to find myself

Doris: There was a period when I lost myself, I lost the person that I am when I became ill, and I feel I've regained some of that but, in regaining some of it, I've picked out the bits that I liked.

Rose: The change is due to actually learning who I am, I've been something else before now.

Abigail: I've spent decades hiding behind drugs and a career and I've had to face up to the actual reality of what is me and learn who is me. So, changing as a person, I am changing.

Leska: I've started to find my identity and I've started to live life again.

Tiffany: I'm finding I'm getting back some of my old personality, the bubbly, loud me.

Donald: People have helped me to reach inside myself and get back to the cheeky little monkey.

7 = Since attending The Haven I have changed as a person because I feel I am getting better

Lucy: I'm feeling better in myself.

Jenny: I think I changed, I can't even really remember when I first came here. I was that unwell. When I first came I was really unwell, lost in my own thoughts really, and I think I obviously have changed a lot, I don't know how.

Tiffany: I'm not as attention seeking and my moods are not as low.

Carl: I'm content with life.

Brunhilda: I'm more down to earth. I used to be off in another galaxy.

4 = Since attending The Haven I have changed as a person because I have more hope for the future

Rose: I look to the future more than I ever did. It exists now.

Jonny: I think, well I know, I've survived it. The other thing is, I think The Haven gives hope to everybody that there's something better in the future. So you're not written off.

3 = Since attending The Haven I have changed as a person because I am able to feel safe

Igor: Coming here makes you feel safe enough to change.

Crystal: I feel safe and relaxed here.

3 = Since attending The Haven I have changed because I have regained my sense of fun

Doris: I am less serious. I have rediscovered my sense of humour and I have rediscovered my ability to make other people laugh.

Brunhilda: I feel I have become light hearted again.

3 = Since attending The Haven I have changed as a person because I am learning to live my life

Leska: I am learning to live again, not just exist.

Chloe: I would like to say that I am certified sane! I don't have a mental health diagnosis at all. I have actually discovered life. It's not even a rediscovery. It's a discovery. Looking at how I am living now, I haven't lived up to now, I have just been surviving. Now I am discovering what it is like to be too busy to ring someone back whereas before I had too much time to think what to do with. I now live a full, active and healthy life and I am thoroughly enjoying it.

2 = Since attending The Haven I have changed as a person because I now want to live

Stony: When I first attended The Haven I didn't like myself, I was wanting to commit suicide. I never though anybody would like me or love me in any way. Now I don't even, I don't want to die.

May: Before The Haven I wanted to die. Now I want to live.

Three clients answered only negatively

Ben: I feel more vulnerable now. I feel like I've got exposed wounds. But everyone here is universally kind so I'm hoping eventually they'll heal.

Phoenix: It's loud and aggressive, that's when for myself I can find it intimidating and more than offensive.

Charles: I don't think I've changed as a person but I feel that I have to take responsibility to be a civilized individual here, for the sake of others obviously and the sake of myself, and obviously my membership for the future.

How would you define recovery? Do you think recovery is frightening?

Of the 60 clients who were asked this question, ten did not respond. The remaining 50 clients who answered this question responded to the concept of recovery in a variety of ways, some defining it in more than one way.

15 = Recovery is an individual journey taken step by step

Doris: I think the journey to recovery is like a road up, a country road that's full of speed bumps and windy corners, and you travel along it and you think, yea you're getting somewhere, then you go over a bump and you get set back a bit, but you have to keep going and eventually you'll get to the end of the road and you'll find another road that goes somewhere that might be less bumpy.

Boris: Recovery for me is just taking it step by step and just seeing where I get to in the end. There's no finishing line for me.

Jonny: I think recovery is part of the journey and it's like change in anybody's life, it's scary unless you continue with the journey. That's probably the most positive thing that The Haven has given us, the chance to continue our journey and to progress, and that's the most important thing, the journey.

Cosmic: I see recovery as not really a game of snakes and ladders, it's just where you are at each day, and it's still a step forward.

Elise: It's an ongoing process, you never actually get there. You are always recovering. For me recovery has been able to actually function on my own, with minimal support, because of the things I've learnt. So, for me, recovery represents now. I'm well into recovery because I've actually developed enough internalized strategy in my brain to cope with things when they go wrong without resorting to emotional crisis. So therefore I would say I am in recovery. But, to be honest, I think everybody's in recovery from the minute they enter the doorway of The Haven, unless they desperately don't want to help themselves, because recovery is a journey and it starts with admitting that you've got the problem to be there in the first place.

Jenny: It's probably the hardest thing I think I have done in my life, and I'm not even there yet. I don't even know if I'm halfway there. I don't even know what 'there' is like. I believe it's a journey, but I don't know if the journey ever ends.

Brunhilda: I think recovery means something different for each person and also I don't think recovery is finite.

15 = Recovery is frightening because of fear of failure

Sally: I'm thinking do I want another job or don't I want another job, am I capable of wanting another job, would I be able to do it, would I have the confidence, or how long would it be before it goes wrong?

Boris: I think recovery is frightening because for so long in my life I had so many people telling me I was never going to come to anything, spend my whole life in hospital. I am petrified that I am going to fail and I am going to prove everyone right. I sit there and I work on my journey to change things with the whole doubt in my head going, what happens if I don't achieve this, what happens if it goes wrong, what happens if I still go backwards?

Masie: Something will happen that sets me about ten steps back and I'm right back at the bottom of the pile again. So therefore I'm frightened to continue on my road to recovery because each time I get a certain way something just knocks me back down again.

Chloe: Success can be frightening. What if I fail?

Harry: It's not the process of recovery that's frightening for me, I'm quite revelling in it actually, it's the thought that I can't guarantee I won't slip back at a future date, that's the thing that's frightening.

Tiffany: I'm frightened of getting well then not being able to work. Like coming off benefits, that's what frightens me most.

Fred: The world I was in before was so black. I was petrified of becoming well and failing every time. Before I wanted to be dead rather than fail again because I just couldn't handle anymore failure.

14 = Recovery is frightening because it's about change and the unknown

Meg: I think basically it's going into the unknown. I do get frightened, but when I see the staff we talk about it, it's shared, and it's reduced in some way.

Elise: I think there's an awful lot of people at The Haven that have lived in a world of inner torment for so long, and have lived a psychiatric based life for so long that to move away from that, even though they don't particularly like the life they have at the moment, but to move away from that and take on something new, with a whole new perspective and everything, it's always going to be scary. It's like moving to another country or a new flat. The change is what's so scary because it's so unpredictable.

Crystal: With recovery you've got to change, and change through life, there's always changes, but if you are the type of person who doesn't know how to change, or has never been taught to change, then it's very hard and you are stuck in that time warp and you have got to find a way of trying to move on.

Alexis: Extremely frightening! We're used to living with what is most familiar to us, it's our routine and it's what goes on day to day, month in, month out.

Ross: It's only natural to fear change, it's the not knowing what's going to happen. That's what we are in fear of.

Eustace: Maybe the process towards it is frightening. Where does it lead you to?

13 = Recovery is frightening because I've always been this way

Ben: Very frightening! Personality disorder is all I've got. If you take that away I've got nothing left.

Sheila: Yes, because it's all I've ever known, is this personality disorder, all this mental illness, ever since I was very young.

Kim: Fucking scary, cos I've never known recovery. I've been in and out the system since 16.

Gemma: I think when you've spent half your life, it's a real struggle. I've found that, since the age of 14 when I started self-harming, over the years I have picked myself up, and now I have gone down again without realising it. In the end you can be so sick and tired of the struggle. You know the will to do it is so hard, it's just so hard. I don't have the energy the strength or the will. Literally last week I tried to end it. I woke up three days later. If I'd had the support, like there is nowadays, with phone lines you can ring, with better understanding of mental health, if that was the case when I was 14. I was in hospital when I was 16. If I was 16 now I would not have gone backwards and forwards into hospital all my life. It would have made my life completely different if I'd had the understanding and not just be called attention seeking because it wasn't, it wasn't.

Igor: Of course it is, psychosis is a nice safe little place.

Leska: It's frightening for me, for the fact that I've spent the last 11 years in hospital, and the thought of people trying to rush me into recovery when I've had it done so many times before, where people have tried to make me recover, where it hasn't been done at my speed.

9 = Recovery can be frightening but desirable

Ian: At the beginning I think it is because it means you have to take a lot more responsibility and sometimes it's scary that people aren't around so much, and you have to deal with things a lot more on your own, but afterwards it makes you proud.

Stony: Yes, but it's good. It is a bit frightening, a bit daunting, but you know, you see so many normal people around and you just want that. I feel like that, people who can go to work and do things for themselves and manage alone.

Curtis: I used to think it was frightening, because it's such a big step, but now I find I'm looking for it, I'm wanting it.

Rose: Yes I think it's frightening, but I also think it's exciting now.

Bling: I think it should be welcomed with open arms.

9 = Recovery is about achieving things in the outside world

Stony: Getting on with life, having a career or a job that you like, and liking yourself.

Doris: I think it's more of a renaissance because I think I've been given a chance now to take stock, and go back to college and do all the things I meant to do before I got ill. I feel I've been given time to reinvent what I really want to do.

Katy: My recovery would be having my family back with me, going back into education, having positive steps forward and regaining my employment status.

Natasha: A more normal life, perhaps even working.

8 = Recovery makes me wonder who I am

Sally: Sometimes you don't know, it takes time to find out who you are and to start to try to change who you are, that takes quite a while.

Abigail: I find recovery is knowing yourself and it's very frightening because you're suddenly finding something that you have never known before and accepting them for who and what they are. I think the frightening thing is that you haven't got that person that's at the end of the line.

Boris: That still petrifies me to this day because what happens if I do recover to the extent where I'm happy and I do like myself and are people that know me going to like me? Am I going to be the same person, am I going to be the person people know now and probably like, because I don't want to be any different. I know I am only the person I am due to where I've come from. I'd like to think that once I had recovered that I was always the same person but there's always that fear inside me that I might not be that person.

Milly: It's frightening for me because I don't know whether, by recovering, I'm going to lose my relationship, because I don't know whether my partner can accept me if I change.

8 = Recovery is about having more realistic goals

Pablo: I asked somebody about recovery some three years ago and she said I'm 99 per cent well and I asked, don't you ever expect to be 100 per cent and she said no. I always thought 100 per cent was going to be my goal and subsequently since then I've realized it's a long process and I don't think 100 per cent is achievable on my old stats. On my new stats I think 100 per cent is more than achievable.

Doris: I think it's bloody hard work. It doesn't just happen, you don't just wake up one morning and think hey, I'm going to be better today. I'm not going to fall down, I'm not, and you have to take it upon yourself and keep doing what you were doing the day before.

Chloe: Everyone has the potential in them to succeed, but it's about taking it each step at a time. It's about setting achievable goals.

Katy: I've got more realistic goals. I've got more realistic about my own boundaries and in my own confidence and it feels, as the weeks go by, I feel safer and safer.

7 = Recovery is about having hope and a concept of a future

Donald: I'm 26 and I've had 24 years of rubbish and it's hard to see a path of recovery but, since I've been coming here, I can see a light somewhere, not sure entirely where it is but I do feel that I could make the next 26 years of my life a bit different.

Emily: I define my recovery, I've got hope now.

Rose: I'm looking to the future, which I would never have done, and I'm hopeful.

6 = Recovery is about having a good quality of life

Ian: Learning to deal with things in a positive way so you can have a good quality of life.

Chloe: I'm talking about success as in how happy and content you are as a person, success in life rather than qualifications and a good job. It's very individual for each of us. It's about breaking out of your own mould that you've made or other people have made for you. It's about breaking out of that mould.

Brunhilda: Is personality disorder an illness or a disability? Because, if it's an illness, there's a possibility of a cure but, if it's a disability then the way to approach it, just as it is of a physical disability, is that it's possible to learn to live a fruitful life.

6 = Recovery is about regaining control and independence

Sheila: Being able to stand on my own two feet, without calling for help every five minutes.

Ross: To regain control. We spend too much time looking for a cure when there is none. We can only learn to live alongside our illnesses by re-thinking the way we think, to retrain the way we go about our daily lives and to learn to use our past experiences to guide us to where we want to be in life rather than carrying on the way we do.

Natasha: Freedom to do what you want without being stopped by disability, getting on with your life in a productive way.

6 = Recovery is having fewer negative symptoms and more feeling of emotions

Fred: Stopping drugs, feeling the emotion and learning from it.

Rose: Recovery for me is being able to feel the real emotions I have run away from for so long.

Meg: No more nightmares.

5 = Recovery is about social interaction and being socially included

Brunhilda: That I am actually part of society at large.

Poppy: Socializing, not just with people from The Haven. Being able to get on buses, go to the supermarket.

Anne: To find the real me inside and to fit in.

2 = Recovery is something you have to want

Doris: All the help in the world is great but you have got to want to get to where you want to be. It's nothing you can be shown. You have just got to get your own fight back.

Charles: Wanting to do it is the main issue. There's nothing wrong with slipping back, it's trying to learn from it.

2 = Recovery is about balance and stability

Cosmic: I'd say that in life everything is striving for equilibrium, to find balance, not being too left or too right, ups or downs. That's how I'd define recovery, to find balance that you once had or to regain what you've never had.

Anne: Stability!

2 = Recovery is about growing up

Lara: Recovery can also be a way of growing up, or finding a new way to grow up again and be at one with yourself and accept yourself as you are.

Bling: I was having an adult conversation, as a normal 33-year-old would. All of a sudden something in my brain said, no that's not alright you effing cow, who do you think you are to judge me, well I'll see you in the effing hospital then when I've taken another overdose, bitch. When I got angry it was how the 13-year-old child, how the teenager would deal with things, instead of what I'd call a normal adult, and it would be something like, well I hope you die in a car crash on your way home, until about three or four years ago, until I got the help that I wanted.

288

2 = Recovery is about regaining control but still having a safety net

Leska: I personally think recovery is still being able to ask for support and say you are struggling but also know that you are getting better and that you don't need the services as much as you did when you were ill.

Cosmic: Well, if I saw a tortoise on its back I think recovery would be putting him the right way up, because that's something he can't do for himself. There's no way a tortoise wanted to get on its back and it was there for circumstances beyond its own control. So, if you help him by putting him back on his feet, and he goes plodding along at his own pace, then who is to say those circumstances won't arise again. So I don't think we can actually confidently say, now I've recovered, you see, but as long as the Tortoise Rescue Centre is still there we'll be alright.

2 = Recovery is not possible for me

Abigail: Yes it's frightening, I can't change and I don't want to change.

Phoenix: I hope that I recover enough to define recovery because I really do not know what it is and where it is or if it's possible anymore. If I was able to do something like cure world poverty I don't think that would ever be enough. I know a good line from a song which goes, 'Dying is easy, it's living that scares me to death,' and I think that maybe says it for me.

Can you say something about hopes, dreams and goals for the future, and whether your vision of this has changed since coming to The Haven?

Of the 60 clients who were asked this question, 46 responded, many answering in a variety of ways.

12 = My hopes, dreams and goals are about education

Rose: My goal is to go to university to get my MA and then take it further.

Boris: I want to go to college and do English and maths with confidence.

Ben: Since coming to The Haven I've had an idea implanted in my head to go back to university and I'm at the stage now where I'm getting the curriculum and believing I might be able to do it.

Alexis: I hope to do mathematics.

Poppy: My goal is to get through college and do my degree.

Katy: My goal is to go back and do my MA. That's my long-term goal.

12 = My hopes, dreams and goals are getting through the day

Stony: I want to get on a bus and breathe at night without panic.

Kim: I want the thoughts of 30 years ago to go away. I should have been in care, I blame my family and my school.

Sally: To be happy, lead a normal life, and come off all meds. I can only cope with one day at a time.

Cosmic: My goal for many years was just getting through the day. I wouldn't know where to start.

Christine: The dream for me is taking one day at a time. Dreams are about finding our destiny and our purpose in life.

Lucy: Trying to feel next week like I've felt this week.

11 = My hopes, dreams and goals have changed and I see the future now

Ian: It has changed. Well, I'm not sure that it's changed, I've always wanted to do something, but now I feel I can actually do it. I have more belief in myself.

Rose: My vision has changed. I didn't even think about the future before I came here. It was as much as I could do to survive today. I hated the thought of tomorrow. I never wanted it to come. I feel I am learning a lot and I would like to put that to some use.

Emily: Do you know what, I never dreamed I could have hopes and dreams and goals for the future until sitting with this lot.

Leska: I actually thought that I have got a future now, it was really bleak before, but it actually looks like there is something now. Now, when I am just unconsciously sitting there, I do find myself wondering and thinking about the future. I don't feel on my own.

Tiffany: I can only say that since I've come to The Haven that I've actually got hopes, goals and dreams, because I've never had them before.

Donald: I never had any before I came here.

8 = My hopes, dreams and goals are about work and having a career

Boris: I would love to train to be a social worker. I want to work with children. I'd rather help children younger, try and steer some kids at a younger age to go out there and chose the life they can.

Elise: For a long time my little aim was to come back and work at The Haven. I do think it would be a very noble thing if we did have people who were former clients coming back to work but, as I've gradually got better, I've discovered there's a whole world of possibilities and employment prospects out there and it doesn't have to all centre around this sort of several walls The Haven is, and I think for me the significant breakthrough is realizing there's other things in life that would be just as enjoyable as coming back to work for The Haven. I'd actually like to go and get a decent job and earn a reasonable amount of money so I can have a nice lifestyle to go with it.

Natasha: I've got high expectations for my future. They are big aims, probably not that easy, but I've got the commitment and I'm quite stubborn, so I hope The Haven can help me get where I want to be.

Jenny: I now want to do my access course and I want to work in care.

7 = My hopes, dreams and goals are now more realistic

Charles: I wasn't being realistic. Rome wasn't built in a day.

Abigail: My hopes and dreams have been totally shattered because of me. I'm learning to accept how things are and I've taken my expectations down, and since I've taken my expectations down everything's gone up.

Calvin: To feel fulfilled, filled up. Not 2.5 children and a garage and a beautiful home. I want to find a way to make a personal goal. Now I don't feel alone. I feel we are in a boat and it's a safe boat.

Katy: Since The Haven my hopes and dreams are becoming a lot more realistic.

5 = My hopes, dreams and goals are about family

Stony: I want to find someone to love me, someone to share my life with, and have a family and things like that, and be in a family.

Pablo: Hope my son nourishes well, and grows up as a balanced kid and I don't, you know, cause him any problems.

Poppy: My dream is to find a nice bloke, get married; have kids and a dog.

4 = My hopes dreams and goals are about changing the system

Jonny: What I want is for all the projects, not just The Haven, to be successful, because the more working together you get the better service you are going to get as a result. I want to educate mental health services.

Harry: I've always been a campaigner for mental health and I want to try and make a difference nationally. My hopes and dreams, they're not dreams anymore because I'm doing it with the Personality Disorder Awareness Program.

4 = My hopes, dreams and goals are about voluntary work

Abigail: To continue with two voluntary jobs.

Alexis: I've recently started helping with the special needs groups at the church.

4 = My hopes, dreams and goals include travel

Masie: My goal is, I'm going to Spain for ten days.

Anne: I haven't been on holiday for probably 12 years, so that was one of my hopes and dreams, to go back abroad. The way I am going on holiday is with somebody I met here.

4 = I have no hopes, dreams and goals

Igor: I've got no dreams apart from nightmares.

Crystal: I've got no hopes, dreams and goals. I feel empty inside.

3 = My hopes, dreams and goals were just to stay alive

Chloe: When I first started coming, when it first opened, my hopes and goals were just to stay alive at that point. Now I want to continue to be happy.

Jenny: Before I came to The Haven I was locked up in a secure unit and my only hopes and goals were to end it all. I've changed everything really, my hopes, dreams and goals, and the whole vision. Before I came to The Haven I used to wake up every day wanting to die, finding a way; thinking of a way that I could harm myself while I was in hospital, trying to trick people into thinking I was okay, trying to sneak things in. That was my life, trying to find a way to actually harm myself, to actually end it all, and now I'm actually going to college!

3 = Hopes, dreams and goals are a risk

Cosmic: At 51 to say that I've recovered is putting a hell of a lot at risk. I'll have to be forced out of this safety net, not that I'm lazy. It's the Government want to get people back to work, and that's what this is, isn't it. I'm getting DLA, rent paid, but I've got a dread of going back to what it was like before. I would overwork, do all the hours under the sun, then come down with depression and alcoholism. I might self-harm then two weeks later get back on my feet and be able to do agency work, work myself to death again. To become a more ethical person, yea, to be able to live in the here and now, to be able to forgive, to be a better Dad, but a career, because of my age, I think I'm over the hill on that one.

Milly: I have a goal but I'm scared I'm not going to fulfil it and will feel a failure.

3 = My hopes, dreams and goals are to work at The Haven

Harry: My goal is to actually work here on bank staff.

Rose: I'd like to study and work within the service.

2 = My hopes, dreams and goals are to show them

Chloe: I guess my goal was just to prove to mental health services that everything is treatable but it's not always in hospital. I think of all those nursing staff, when I was in high secure hospital, I'm now in employment. I'm in my own flat. They would never even envision that happening. And I think I've shown it to them, you know.

Boris: I have one goal I know I'll achieve and that's to turn around and say to all the fucking twats that have fucked up my life and say, fuck you, I've won, you've lost. If I can't achieve anything else in my life that's what I want to achieve and will achieve.

2 = My hopes, dreams and goals are to live in the now

Brunhilda: I think for most of my life I've had no direction and I've ended up doing all sorts of weird and wonderful stuff. There's a kind of certain way of looking at life which says hopes are illusions, it takes you out of the present and the whole point is to live in the present. My vision of the future has changed since coming to The Haven because, when I first came, I thought I had absolutely no future except endurance. So I feel more positive about the future, but I don't really have many goals or dreams. I'm much more able to live in the present and to enjoy the present as well sometimes. I quite often enjoy the present.

1 = My hopes, dreams and goals are that The Haven continues to be here

Pablo: I hope The Haven remains there to hand-hold me on my bad days, not many. I know it's a lot to ask, but that's the truth of it.

1 = My hopes, dreams and goals are to find me

Anne: My dream has always been to find the real me inside and I think The Haven is starting to help me to find the real true me. One of my hopes and dreams was to fit in, into this world, and being at The Haven I think I've finally started to fit in.

1 = I think it is important to have hopes, dreams and goals

Bling: It's good to have goals, it's important to have goals.

What else do you feel The Haven could do to support you in recovery?

Forty-eight clients were asked this question and 38 responded, some giving more than one answer.

10 = Providing outreach support would help my recovery

Elise: One of the ways that recovery can be supported is if people are actually helping you live lives in the actual community, outside the four walls that are The Haven, maybe helping people have new flat starts and that kind of thing. If people actually get to the point where they have recovered to the extent that they want to go back to work then maybe there can be some support package drawn up.

Leska: I have had a baby and I am feeling quite isolated and it's so hard to kind of still stay positive when you haven't got the support that helps you along with that and keeps you afloat.

Natasha: Self-esteem and confidence, it's quite a major issue, I am getting some one-to-one support in going to college, someone's going to college with me. Going to college is quite a big deal.

Fred: I need a little bit of help with moving.

Poppy: I do feel I need outreach work for when I'm at home.

8 = The Haven is already doing all it can to support me in recovery

Sheila: I think they are doing all they can.

Curtis: I don't think they can do any more than they are now.

Meg: I genuinely feel that sufficient is being done by the staff, community and the people here.

Sally: They are doing as much as they can at the moment, you can't ask for no more.

6 = The Haven staying as it is would support my recovery

Pablo: It's in place really, it's well thought out. I hope it doesn't get institutionalized.

Phoenix: I think quality, not necessarily quantity, is important in that you do so much here and so much that is amazing, and it would be awful if that were to be diluted and sort of try and stretch too far.

Bling: What they are doing is absolutely brilliant and they don't need to change.

5 = Tackling stigma and educating the outside world would support my recovery

Christine: We need to educate.

Calvin: I think to let some of the naïve world, the outside world, sort of like people from the A&E Department, they need to be addressed, they need to come along and make an effort to see what goes on, and the police who do 136s.

Jenny: I just want to do something. I just want to stop this whole stigma around it and I think getting it out into the media, because they are the ones who are portraying it so badly, that we are all going out and killing people. I just think this thing, like Personality+, is going to be really good. I think if we can actually get out there and keep on doing these conferences and everything so people are aware that we are not all mad.

5 = The Haven can support my recovery just by being there

Ian: It's just knowing it's there.

Eustace: Just be here.

Charles: Keeping me in a safe place within myself and continuing to do so and just keep coming and using the place.

4 = The Haven would support my recovery by having more outings

Anne: More days out in the summer.

Ross: Send us all on a holiday.

3 = The Haven would support my recovery by having a mini bus

Igor: Get a mini bus.

Wilf: We'll have to get a mini bus.

2 = The Haven can support my recovery by sticking to policies and boundaries

Doris: Basic things like sticking to policies would be useful, so everyone knows where they are at, not just useful for my personal recovery. We all do things that are socially unacceptable but it is really better to make them a little less acceptable, like they are in the big wide world.

Boris: I suppose the biggest issue for me would have to be the boundaries of The Haven, and the policies need to be kept because to aid someone's recovery you need boundaries and that's what so many people lack.

2 = The Haven would support my recovery by giving me more knowledge

Crystal: I'd like to learn a lot more knowledge about The Haven and what goes on here, information and knowledge.

Brunhilda: I like the idea of, I think it's called transitional recovery, or something like that, and I'd like to know more about it.

2 = The Haven would support my recovery by giving me prompts when needed

Doris: A kick up the arse when needed.

Poppy: A kick up the backside.

1 = The Haven would support my recovery by concentrating on those making progress

Cosmic: The staff could be more accessible and stop spending all their time on attention seekers and people that just go home, get wrecked and come back, and are on that cycle.

1 = The Haven can support me by providing more help to get people to recovery

Stony: I think they are doing enough for people who want to be in recovery, maybe they should do more in supporting people to get to that stage.

1 = The Haven would support my recovery by providing support for carers

Harry: The other thing is I'd like to see something for carers. Carers get forgotten. Our carers need support as well.

1 = The Haven would support my recovery by helping me get voluntary work

Tiffany: The Haven should help us get voluntary work.

1 = The Haven would support my recovery by having the Pat Dog every day

Wilf: Meg every day.

1 = The Haven would support my recovery by having faith in me

Ross: Have faith in me. Instil faith.

1 = The Haven would support my recovery by linking clinical work with recovery and goals

Brunhilda: I think at some point in the focused one-to-ones I could be helped to look at questions 10 and 11.

Have you got anything more to add?

Twenty-four clients had something more to add and three had more than one thing to add.

7 = I would like to say thank you to The Haven

Jenny: Thank The Haven for helping me get this far, which I never thought I'd be able to do. To tell the truth I didn't even want to come here at first. I'm so glad I decided to try and actually get some help.

Anne: I'd just like to thank The Haven for teaching me not to run away from everything all the time, but actually stay and face what the problems are.

Fred: Can I give an apology here. When I was ill I was shouting my head off and swearing at the staff because I thought they were demons. I didn't do that meaning to hurt or be nasty to anyone. I really didn't know what I was doing or saying. So, whoever was on that day, thanks, you know, for not sending me away.

Leska: Since I've come to The Haven I have never met such a wonderful bunch of people, and staff especially, and the kindness and everything that you can imagine really, that a lot of people haven't had, it's just out of this world and, if it's okay, I would just like to add a great big thank you, and I hope this is the way it will always stay.

4 = I would like to say that The Haven is a wonderful service

Curtis: I love The Haven, I think it's a wonderful place, a wonderful project, and long may it continue.

Daniel: I'd like to say to all staff members at The Haven that they are doing a brilliant job.

3 = The Haven is unlike any other service I have known

Cosmic: This is the most effective system of care I've ever seen.

Sheila: After a lifetime of using mental institutions The Haven's the only place that accepts you as you are and doesn't try to dictate to you. They are not critical and are just accepting.

2 = The Haven needs to keep track of community members that aren't around

Daniel: Sometimes a client gets sectioned and you don't know about it, no one knows do they.

Harry: I think if someone's not been in, it would be rather nice if a staff member could keep a note of the fact, just making a quick call to make sure that person is okay.

2 = The Haven involves us in research and policies

Harry: Can I just say that it's really important, the fact that The Haven has included us in the research, and I feel very privileged to have been able to be in that group.

Brunhilda: I think it's great the way clients take such a part in research and setting parameters and policies.

1 = There are some things I would change about how The Haven is run

Pablo: I'm disappointed with the way staff are selected. I wouldn't choose some of the staff we have here at initial interview. I'd choose them after I'd seen what they are. It does bother me that other people would like to give up smoking and can't. They're not being given the opportunity to stop because they are being pressured into coming for a fag. I'd like results from some groups sometimes, like the gardening group, it would be nice for their plans to be published on the wall for a week or two before, so everyone can go, cor that's a good idea, or, what about that. To end on a positive note, I am proud of it, I feel good about it, I like the people here and I like the staff, and I like what goes on. I've got no regrets about what I've just said.

1 = The Haven has improved

Stony: I think The Haven's doing better now, with the behavioural policy in place, and the fact that they have a move-on group, the transitional recovery group.

1 = The Haven Pat Dog is great

Doris: The other group I love, or part of the group that I enjoy most is when Meg the Pat Dog comes in because I bring my puppy in and we all go for a big hairy walk around hilly fields and they all love it.

1 = The Haven should be more honest

Tom: I think the staff and the clients should be more honest, I do. When things go wrong it shouldn't take so long to sort out because the honesty does affect each one of us.

1 = The substance misuse support group is very helpful

Rose: The substance misuse group is extremely helpful.

1 = Dependency on The Haven should be discouraged in a gentle way

Elise: I think, fundamentally, people with PD need a certain amount of love and care and TLC and pampering and I think The Haven's taken that well on board and has supplied that, where other statutory units have failed dismally. I do think it's very easy to pour out the love and concern and that's so important because so many people haven't had that, but then I think there's a danger that that then becomes an emotional crutch and people don't particularly want to move on. That dependency shouldn't be fostered; it should be actively discouraged in a very gentle way. The program of activities that runs needs to be constantly developed towards developing life skills for people so that, at the end of the day, they can actually go out and live that life.

1 = Last Christmas at The Haven was the best I ever had

Cosmic: Last Christmas was the best Christmas I ever had, at The Haven. There was more of a family atmosphere here than I've ever had with my family.

1 = The Haven has become my family

Tiffany: I just feel The Haven have become my family, the family that I lost.

1 = If The Haven is used in the right way it works

Charles: It's a good place you know, use it, don't abuse it, and it will work for you.

Appendix VIII Findings from Family and Carer Questions

Do you think the term 'carer' is appropriate? If not, do you feel another term would be better?

Six family members or carers were asked this question and five responded, two responding in more than one way.

4 = The term 'carer' has practical uses in relation to professional bodies

Sammy: There are new laws coming in, in respect of carers, where, if you suddenly do away with the term, human resources, all of these departments won't actually accept. There are a lot of new things carers are getting, so we've got to be careful about changing terms.

Dinah: I've had to use the word carer recently but it was to my employers to explain why I might need time off and it needs to be a word that they understand the meaning of and that's why I used the word carer.

Tony: It does help to throw that word in if you are trying to chase up prescriptions, speak to a chemist, whereas in those areas the word carer does come in handy.

Rob: We did decide that we needed to use the term when talking to professionals.

2 = The term carer is acceptable

Alex: I can't think of another term that would be more appropriate, personally.

Sammy: I have no objection to it.

2 = A prefix of 'informal' or 'family carer' could make the term clearer

Sammy: Quite often you have to preface it with the word informal carer, because we are not carers supplied by the County Council. A lot of professionals actually think carer means someone who is a paid professional. So you don't get confused with people who work for care agencies, just to differentiate between us who are very professional and the so-called professionals!

Tony: What about suggesting something on say, family carer, to make it more specific. We are supporting a relative or a loved one, rather than carer, sounds sort of very formal doesn't it, but if you throw the family in front of it.

1 = A family member does not mean a carer

Rob: I don't like the term carer. I don't do anything different because of who she is, I'm just a husband; you're adding something that's already there.

Do you feel The Haven has helped the person you support? If yes, how? If no, what would you like The Haven to do for them?

Six family members or carers were asked this question and all responded.

4 = The Haven has provided support that has been very helpful

Alex: I feel, definitely, it's helped my daughter. It's somewhere safe for her to come, somewhere without any bad memories. She's got friends here, I think she feels even the staff are her friends as well, and I just feel that she feels that it's more her home now. This place has taken the place of her home, although that's a very hard thing to accept as her Mum, but I do thank you. Her communication skills, she can talk to us as a family now, having somewhere to go when she feels things are getting on top of her and you guys seem to have time and patience, and the understanding and reassurance and you've gained the trust I think, which is one of the things when people come out of hospital, or before they come here, that they haven't got trust in anything. I mean the people that love and care for them, not in the mental health system, they don't trust anyone. But when they come here it's a gradual trust in people. They don't feel they are going to be let down and that's a big positive and then they gradually can begin even to trust themselves to do things and take responsibility. But that only comes when they begin to trust other people, and then other people begin to trust them.

Sarah: I have to say that I just think The Haven is just a calm, happy, just a caring place. To be honest I found the hospital a hustle and bustle, and just total chaos. I personally feel that, total chaos, and nobody really, I don't know how to explain it really, nobody really, I'm sure they are trying to help, but I have reservations on that, because they just did not help my son at all, and if I asked for help I don't really think I got any help at all. I can honestly say I got nowhere, absolutely nowhere. I have to say, I might have a tear in a minute, I have to say that The Haven is just, it's a wonderful place really. I really mean that.

Rob: She has been dealing with things for a long time and, since the diagnosis, and getting the help, she has got much, much better, and coming, she doesn't just come if she's in crisis, she comes and has a bed which she arranges in advance and uses that, and she really does work hard while she's here, talking and making use of everything that's here. She's doing things at home she wouldn't do before. Gradually it kind of sinks in, and that helps in your relationship, because once you start understanding what the problem is then you can start to work towards a better way of carrying on, mustn't say cure must we! It does work; well it works for my wife. It's keeping her alive, I don't think she would be alive without The Haven. She tried to kill herself desperately under the care of the hospital and previous regimes. It's the right treatment, the right care, and it's obviously working. I'm fortunate enough to see how similar projects have helped their clients and it just didn't compare. I can see it's not right for a lot of other people there, it's depressing; it's horrible. Promise to be around forever.

Sammy: I think it's been absolutely useful her being here, my wife. It's actually given her motivation that for many years prior to coming here, that we tried to get her to get up and do things. Coming here has given that to her and the ongoing support, no matter how many times a week you come, there is a plan and people phone her which has given her support outside of when she's here. But to actually see her wanting to do different things and actually doing different things indoors now is far better. It's the motivation we've been trying to give her for years. But to pick up on what Rob was saying, and relate it directly back to The Haven; The Haven serves a specialist community in a very specialist way. The hospitals and the community mental health teams, their only speciality is mental health, where The Haven is catering for a group of people and a limited number so, actually, you can work far better with those individuals and be more focused, so we certainly don't want it to go away.

1 = My partner doesn't always use The Haven

Dinah: It's coping skills that we need and those are the strategies I hope The Haven will give to my partner. My partner's a bit naughty in that I will actually wave her goodbye because she's going to The Haven, but it's only sort of a few weeks later that I discover she's not going. So I've got a continuing problem, she's not coping very well at the moment, and now I know she's not coming in. My partner has a ferocious temper and aggressive behaviours, and it's frightening, I find it very frightening, and for years I've put up with it, frightened in my own house, when she goes into one. I can now say, 'You are frightening me; you will leave now,' and she has to go. We get these suicide attempts and we've been to hospital numerous times. I've run out of sympathy, quite frankly, because the first time it's, 'Oh my God,' you know, the second times it's, 'Oh,' the third time it's, 'Not again.' I'm not going to play the game anymore. I'm being pushed to a point that I'm having my strings pulled and I can't; I can't cope with all that manipulation that's being put on me.

1 = My family member has worsened since receiving the diagnosis

Tony: In times of crisis it's very helpful but I've found with my Mum, since she's had the diagnosis, the title, she has completely given in to it. Whereas prior to that she used to fight, she used to try and do things to rationalize things, to work through them, whereas I've found, since she's had the personality disorder diagnosis she, I know it sounds hard, but she almost uses it as an excuse, 'I'm in crisis, I'm not going to deal with this, I've got a personality disorder,' and gives up, and never actually challenges what it is that's causing the problem. The biggest problem with my Mum is drug-induced. She's quite a bad drug addict, cannabis, which does encourage psychosis anyway, and drug-induced psychosis if it's used an awful lot. I have been telling my Mum for a couple of years now; the drugs have got to go for her to improve. As far as I'm aware Mum's making no effort to stop. She was stoned on Wednesday before her three children and her grandson turned up. I'm afraid that I'm at the end of my tether because of drugs and, as far as I'm concerned, are keeping my Mum ill and she doesn't seem prepared to let it go. So, if you can help her in that aspect that might help. I'm also aware my Mum's sold drugs, I'm really concerned; I caught my Mum out Christmas time drug dealing to children. There's a 16-year-old child in my house at the moment, so any advice you're giving to handle it, or anything I can find out. Drugs are a huge issue. What I've tried to do for my Mum is also issue an ultimatum, 'It's your drugs or your children or your grandchild.' My auntie hung herself a couple of years ago, which is a very huge issue, because I was very close to my auntie, and with my Mum's self-harm and suicide attempts I am terrified to lose another one. So if I withdraw, although it's tough love, is that going to happen again?

Do you feel The Haven involves you in the care offered to the person you support? If yes, how? If no, what would you like The Haven to do to improve this?

Six family members or carers were asked this question and five responded, some answering in more than one way.

3 = The Haven has provided an acceptable level of involvement

Sammy: I think it is fair to say that The Haven is here primarily to support the client. I would say it doesn't support me directly; it does indirectly by the fact that it supports the client.

Rob: It's about the right level I think, for me. I haven't been refused an answer.

Alex: Every time I've contacted they've always been very supportive.

2 = I don't want too much involvement

Rob: I don't get dragged into anything. I don't want to get dragged into it. If I want to phone anyone and talk to anyone there's never been a problem but, as I say, I don't really think you contact me a lot. I suppose, in theory, I just hand her over to you, you know, just drop-you-off, there you go, carry on and come home when you've had your session.

Dinah: I'm not sure I want to be involved in the care of my partner's recovery, and to qualify that it is my partner who doesn't have the ability to cope with life, and if you give her a crutch, which is me, she uses it. I'm completely capable and I end up making all her phone calls, or could I do this, could I do that. She's got to cope on her own, and learn strategies and own her problems and deal with them.

1 = I am very careful not to shatter trust by speaking directly to The Haven

Alex: If I am a bit worried about my daughter, and I'm going away for a week and she's not coming, then I think I would tend to talk to her CPN (community psychiatric nurse) who would then relay the information to you. The reason I do that is there have been times when my daughter alienates the family, cuts us off and not wanted us to know anything. Then it puts you in a precarious position because I feel it is important that she knows she can always come to you no matter what and that you are never going to tell us anything that she doesn't want us to know. I don't feel that I would pick up the phone and ask you anything that might jeopardize how my daughter feels about you. This is her haven, this is her one place that nobody ever lets her down and I can actually turn around and say to my daughter, no I haven't spoken to The Haven, I haven't told them anything, and I won't be lying.

1 = I would like The Haven to get my side of the story

Tony: My Mum's a compulsive liar; it's part of her. If Mum's got a problem with me talk to me because she invents things, and the first I know about it is when I get phone calls from friends of my Mum. Perhaps contact with the family, ask our side of things that are actually happening perhaps, to try to get to the root of it, because obviously my Mum is in crisis for a reason, and rather than dealing with the reason she's making one up. Perhaps to be involved on a quiet level, an update of what is going on perhaps on the family side of things, and as much or what you can say of what's going on my Mum's side. My Mum would, if I'm there all the time, lean on me and it's exhausting, and my back aches through carrying the weight. But to be involved like I say would help her, but not too much in the foreground, to find her own two feet. A member of staff I spoke to, I appreciated it so much at that particular time. When I have had contact it has been very helpful.

1 = Set up an informal carers' group at The Haven

Sammy: I would like to see some kind of informal carers' group run through The Haven.

Research shows that carers often experience difficulties in caring. Do you think this statement is correct and in which way do you think the role affects carers?

Six family members or carers were asked this question and five responded directly to the question; however, participants felt that there were relevant responses to this concept implicit in statements made in response to other questions.

5 = The caring role can impact negatively, cause stress and have an effect on one's own mental health

Dinah: Because they know how to push our buttons, don't they, to get themselves back to the centre of attention.

Alex: The answer is yes, there are difficulties in being a carer, and one of the ways it affects carers is their own mental health, because I think when the person you are caring for is extremely low, then you can't help it but, you know, it's very difficult to keep on top of it and keep bouncy yourself. It's very easy to start going down that slippery lane yourself and ending up ill, and then it's harder for the person to bounce back again, because you're low, and it's just a vicious circle, becomes a vicious circle and you don't know who's bloody most depressed in the end, the carer or the person.

Rob: I used to explode. You say depressed, I used to call it having the hump! And my hump was for a reason, you know, the person I love is hurting the person I love, and that gives me the hump, and wasting a lot of time in A&E, I hate hospitals, you know, hanging around wasting time, and I would explain exactly why I've got the hump, being you know, down, depressed, whatever.

Sarah: At one stage, with my son, it was just like a rollercoaster, and I had family members saying to me, 'Just let him get on with It,' you know, because my son would always ring me, and I would be going up to the hospital picking him up, or whatever, ambulances and all sorts, and I suppose as a Mum I couldn't not go. I was bombarded with, you know, daughters, brothers, husbands, 'You shouldn't be doing this,' and trying to explain to them the little I knew then. It's off-loaded so much from my shoulders; I have to say, because I think I was the one that went through most of it with my son.

Sammy: Being a carer's a very easy job when things are running very smoothly, but when they dip, for the person you care for, they become very stressful. So, in getting the hump, feeling depressed, feeling low, but the person you care for it plateaus off and starts coming up the other side, and levels off again, but the stress as far as I'm concerned, for the person who's caring, carries on for a longer period of time than it does for the person who's plateaued off because, what you are then starting to look for is, has it actually done the plateauing off? Or is it just about to do this again? So, the person who's been down, feeling suicidal, doing things, hearing things, whatever, goes away, they plateau off, maybe a week, ten days, two weeks, two months, whatever, but for the carer that experience you've got to add another per cent of time on to that when you are still in a stressed state.

Are there ways in which you feel you could be supported by The Haven in your role?

Six family members or carers were asked this question and one responded directly to the question, in two ways, however, participants felt that there were relevant responses to this concept implicit in statements made in response to other questions.

1 = Information and knowledge about personality disorder would help me

Sarah: I don't understand, you know. I'm a bit green really, in this.

1 = A stay, for my family member, in a respite bed at The Haven helps me

Sarah: That was just amazing really. I knew that I could probably go to sleep and that he was going to be okay and safe.

Do you feel that the person you support has changed since attending The Haven?

Six family members or carers were asked this question and four responded directly to the question, three in more than one way; however, participants felt that there were relevant responses to this concept implicit in statements made in response to other questions.

3 = The person I support has changed for the better

Sammy: Yes, for the better.

Alex: Oh definitely positive – yea.

Rob: Yes, without a doubt. She's coping with this move.

3 = The behaviour of the person I support has changed since attending The Haven

Rob: The person hasn't changed, the behaviour has changed.

Alex: Yes, I agree with that, the person hasn't changed, the behaviour has changed.

Tony: I think the only positive thing is perhaps the self-harm and suicide attempts aren't as frequent.

1 = The person I support is more motivated since attending The Haven

Sammy: A lot more motivation, getting up and doing things.

1 = The communication of the person I support has improved since attending The Haven

Alex: Her communication skills are definitely a lot better since she's been coming here.

Do you have hope about the future in relation to the person you support?

Six family members or carers were asked this question and five responded.

4 = Yes I have hope about the future in relation to the person I support, but with some reservations or fears

Rob: Yes, I've got hope but I always worry about The Haven being there. That it'll grow. Your community has a size at the moment that obviously works. I hope she can get better and better, but life at the moment's not bad, you know, touch wood. It's a certain level of living, not just comfortable, happy, you know, some of the time, laughter.

Sammy: Yes, I do have hope for the future. I have a bit of a concern the person I care for expressed to me. What happens if The Haven sort of considers that she has got to a point where they can't help her anymore? The problem is what she's worried about is if she's been under mental health services for 30 years. I think this is the fear of, 'Well everyone perceives that I'm, you know, I don't need this anymore?'

Sarah: I would like to say that we do seem to be, at this present time anyway, he is very much better.

Alex: Yes, I have never given up hope, ever, and recently, for the last six months I've had more hopes than ever. My daughter's turning the corner and able to live a fairly normal life, as normal as she can. I would say she seems better in herself, more able to perform the normal things that people do. I think it is scary hoping. I think we are all frightened to hope too much.

1 = No, I can't invest any more hope

Tony: No, I'm so sorry, until my Mum puts drugs out of her life, no, none whatsoever. I'd love to be positive and, to be honest with you; it's hurt so much over the years I can't invest any more hope in my Mum. I'm sorry, that sounds awful, very callous and mean. Social services have been involved with my younger brothers and drugs have been an issue for both my brothers from the age of 16. Mum's still blatantly open and obvious about her drug taking and, unfortunately, I nearly lost one of my brothers before Christmas and, after seeing your son almost die from an accident that was because of drugs, if that's not an incentive to start doing things right I don't think there will ever be an incentive that's enough, so, my hope's gone.

How would you define recovery?

Six family members or carers were asked this question and four responded, one in more than one way.

3 = Recovery is a journey individual to the person

Sammy: Not the way most professionals do. Recovery is an individual thing. It is not necessarily, as a lot of professionals will lead you to believe, about getting a job. At the end of the day, for some people, it might just be getting out of the house for the first time in five years. It's an individual thing; it isn't a model, although some people try to tell you it is. It's a concept and it's an individual concept. It's not about government targets of getting a million people off of incapacity benefit. It's about a journey that somebody takes, and The Haven is assisting people in making that journey, some will fall back, some will go forward, but it's nothing that is actually, for me, specific. It's a totally individual thing for each person. I cringe when people say the Recovery Model; there is no Recovery Model, there is no such thing, it's individual for everybody. Recovery is a goal for the individual and little steps along the way. But whether they will ever be recovered is a totally different thing altogether. You will never, ever know until you get there. I get annoyed by general services that have an end goal that recovery is work. Stand the ministers up in front of me and I will shoot and gun them down because they haven't got a clue what they are talking about. I get totally cheesed off by some of these people with power, this idea of getting everyone back to work. A particular minister actually said one thing at a meeting I was at. A hundred thousand people the Prime Minister keeps on talking about, it's rubbish. What we need to be doing is trying to stop future generations falling into the big black hole that we are in today because 90,000 of those 100,000 will still be claiming benefits in ten years' time. I suppose that the first bit of sense I've heard is actually admitting that the targets are a load of rubbish; I know they are rubbish. You are not going to achieve getting all those people back to work.

Dinah: I don't think recovery will ever be a position where you are declared well and put all this behind us, it won't be like that. I think this is going to be one of those things that will go through my partner's life forever and that certain trigger points, crisis points, certain issues will set her off again and we'll take a step back and there'll be times when we take a few steps forward and life's comparatively easy. How I define recovery for my partner is that she has her own life, and she feels capable of doing things outside, meeting friends, having a bit of a social life, where I'm not standing behind her propping her up or anything, and she has a little bit of a life of her own, and doing the shopping without having a major panic, that's recovery, it's not a set definition. She's never going to hold a job down in a million years. I think my partner's always going to be happy to do a bit of farming, or looking after animals, a much easier life, where the demands are there but in a different way. I think that will be recovery.

Rob: I just think it's the individual thing. One thing I did think is there's no definition, but while they are moving forward they're in a state of recovery. If they keep moving that's good.

1 = Recovery is about having a more normal life but, for a young person, there may be more pressures

Alex: Just having the ability to live a fairly normal life and be happy in themselves. Perhaps it's different for different ages. I think if you are a young person then you obviously want to do more. So it's harder, I don't really know. I think, unlike you guys with your wives, you can shelter them from a certain amount of things, I think. If you keep them well they plateau. I'm looking at my daughter, she wants to go to college, she wants to do this, she wants to do that, when she's feeling well, and I think to myself, all those things are extra pressures on her that nobody can take away. When it's exam time, or when she's going to college every day, there's not anyone who will say, Oh I will do that for you, is there. It's something she's got to do for herself, she's got to go down that road.

1 = Recovery is seeing again the person I used to know

Dinah: Another part of recovery which I suppose is that I get glimpses of my old partner. There are times when you recognize the woman you loved, you fell in love with, that sparkly, exciting, dynamic, creative individual who attracted you in the first place, and I wasn't attracted to the depressed, crying, cutting, tablet nibbling individual that I live with. To see what I saw originally, through all that, that's part of recovery, and I like to be with her, I like to spend time with her, she's fun.

How would you know that the person you are supporting is making progress in their recovery?

Six family members or carers were asked this question and all six responded.

3 = The person I support has hope

Rob: I think hope. They have hope, because I know with my wife, she didn't want to be around, so there was no tomorrow and now she has hope. She can see the future.

Sarah: They can see light at the end of the tunnel, they can see a bit of future really.

Sammy: The periods of wellness are greater than the periods of illness. Probably 18, 20 years ago there was absolutely no hope; they had no hope at all. We've had the conversation more than once, 'Yes I am glad I am now alive, where 20, 25 years ago I wasn't happy that I was alive. I want to be alive now, I want to be well. I want to carry on living.'

2 = The person I support is, or would be, happy

Alex: They are happier in themselves, and they view the world differently, they have the ability to consider other people, not just themselves.

Dinah: If they're happy, I'm happy.

1 = The person I support would be working again

Tony: You see my Mum used to, she used to be in a good job, and I don't understand what happened. We had a series of difficult things happen, but then we've always had a series of difficult things in my 26 years of life, if you go back through our family history we've had physical abuse, sexual abuse, through my family, children given away, so we've had so much stuff going on. What I don't understand is how she functioned for so long. It wasn't until she came back to Colchester, and it all went wrong. So why have we got this shell of the person we had before, 'Why have you bothered coming back because you are no good to anybody?' We've always had hiccups, something, dramas, whatever, from word go. So why now, over the last two or three years has she given in to it, because like I say she always managed to brush herself off.

What else do you feel The Haven could do to help you and the person you support in their recovery?

Six family members or carers were asked this question and three responded.

3 = Ensure that The Haven gets its funding and stays here

Dinah: I do fear for the funding. I've never had any dealings with mental health until I met my partner and I'm appalled that how I see it as the Cinderella subject in the health service and disgusted at the way any cuts come down on the mental health side first. You continue to get your funding and I know it's difficult in this economic climate. I've seen the economics cut £10,000 where it would save you £50,000 later.

Rob: I still worry but I have seen some wonderful figures about how much money it saves. Just keep going.

Sarah: I would just say let's hope it carries on being here.

Have you got anything more to add?

Six family members or carers were asked this question and four responded.

3 = It really helps family members and carers to talk to each other

Alex: The chats that we have as carers, I think we can learn a lot from each other because we are discussing something with somebody else who knows where you are coming from and that just makes a difference. It's good for us all to see a different side isn't it.

Sarah: Yes, totally, you are right, my first time here, I didn't have any support before, and listening to everybody.

Rob: I've got something from you too, because you have an entirely different perspective, and we had a daughter last time; different ways of looking at the same thing.

1 = Don't let The Haven get too big and keep treating everyone as the individual they are

Sammy: There are different labels, but within the label everyone is still an individual and that's what gets lost in the majority of services that isn't lost here. It would be if you tried to double your capacity. What's wrong with general services is they are trying to support everyone as best they can, and for some they do it very well, for some they do it very, very badly, but for the majority of people they just do it averagely. Here, for 90 per cent of your clients it's an individual and absolute positive; it 'aint going to be for a 100 per cent of people because nothing fits everybody.

Appendix IX Service Savings Analysis 2006 and 2013

Table A9.1 The Haven's Impact on Use of NHS and Community Services

Service savings analysis	Data Collected by The Haven for the first 50 registered clients in 2006			Data collected by The Haven for the last 50 registered clients in 2013		
	Annual average use over 2 years prior	Annual average use since attending The Haven	% Reduction	Annual average use over 2 years prior	Annual average use since attending The Haven	% Reduction
Psychiatric inpatient admissions	55	8	85.50	33	6	81.82
Section 136s (No. of times)	43	18	58.10	29	3	89.66
Other sections (No. of times)	11	4	63.60	12	1	91.67
Use of crisis team	187	42	77.50	47	9	80.85
Use of community mental health team	36	14	61.10	23	10	56.52
Use of hospital day care services	32	14	56.30	29	2	93.10
Use of NERIL (Helpline)	1264	317	74.92	449	192	57.24
Use of eating disorder services	56	14	75.00	7	0	100.00

Psychological/counselling not at specialist service	30	21	30.00	31	6	80.65
Use of GP	611	459	24.90	607	398	34.43
Use of A&E	141	77	45.40	89	47	46.89
General hospital admissions	47	37	21.30	37	21	43.24
Children's social services	14	6	57.10	15	12	20.00
Housing/homeless	11	2	81.80	12	5	58.33
Police/probation/prison	13	2	84.60	14	7	50.00
Debt agencies	7	1	85.70	13	5	61.54
Use of external advocacy services	39	11	71.80	9	1	88.89

References

Abley, S. (2014) *Personality Disorder Services in North East Essex.* Colchester: Enable East.

Adlam, J, Aiyegbusi, A., Kleinot, P. Motz, A. and Scanlon, C. (eds) (2012) *The Therapeutic Milieu under Fire.* London: Jessica Kingsley Publishers.

Adshed, G. and Jacob, C. (2009) *Personality Disorder: The Definitive Reader.* London: Jessica Kingsley Publishers.

Aiyegbusi, A. and Norton, K. (2009) 'Modern Milieus: Psychiatric Inpatient Treatment in the Twenty-First Century.' In I. Norman and I. Ryrie, (eds) *The Art and Science of Mental Health Nursing,* 2nd edn. Maidenhead: Open University Press.

Allen, J.G., Fonagy, P. and Bateman, A. (2006) *Mentalizing in Clinical Practice.* Arlington: American Psychiatric Publishing.

Allott, P., Loganathan, L. and Fulford, K.W.M. (2003) 'Discovering hope for recovery from a British perspective.' *Canadian Journal of Community Mental Health 3,* p.21.

Alwin, N., Blackburn, R., Davidson, K., Hilton, M., Logan, C. and Shine, J. (2006) *Understanding Personality Disorder: A Report by the British Psychological Society.* London: British Psychological Society.

American Psychiatric Association (2005) *Position Statement on Use of the Concept of Recovery.* APA Official Actions: Approved by the Assembly, May 2005. Approved by the Board of Trustees, July 2005.

Anthony, W.A. (1993) 'Recovery from mental illness: the guiding vision of the mental health service system in the 1990s.' *Psychosocial Rehabilitation Journal 16,* 11–23.

Appleby, J. (2013) *Spending on Health and Social Care Over the Next 50 Years. Why Think Long Term?* London: The Kings Fund.

Attar, F. (1984) *The Conference of the Birds.* London: Penguin.

Bannister, P., Burman, E., Parker, I., Taylor, M. and Tindall, C. (1994) *Qualitative Methods in Psychology: A Research Guide.* Buckingham: Open University Press.

Bartlett, F. (1932) *Remembering.* Cambridge. Cambridge University Press.

Bateman, A. and Fonagy, P. (2004) 'Mentalization-based treatment of BPD.' *Journal of Personality Disorders 18,* 1, 36–51.

Bateman, A. and Fonagy, P. (2008) '8-year follow-up of patients treated for borderline personality disorder: Mentalization-based treatment versus treatment as usual.' *American Journal of Psychiatry in Advance, March,* 1–7.

Bateman, A. and Tyrer, P. (2004) 'Psychological treatment for personality disorders.' *Advances in Psychiatric Treatment 10,* 378–388.

BBC (2010) *A Centre in Colchester, which treats people with personality disorders, has set up an appeal.* BBC Look East Television News, 26th January 2010.

BBC (2014) *Access to Work Programme 'denying disabled chance to work'.* BBC Television News, 30 October 2014.

Beresford, P. (2013) *From Personal and Individual Problems to Social Understanding.* Paper to the Finnish User Involvement Conference: There is no recovery without social inclusion. Lahti, 1 October 13.

Beresford, P. and Wallcraft, J. (1997) 'Psychiatric System Survivors and Emancipatory Research: Issues, Overlaps and Differences.' In C. Barnes and G. Mercer (eds.) *Doing Disability Research.* Leeds: The Disability Press.

Bettleheim, B. (1950) *Love is Not Enough.* New York: The Free Press.

Bettleheim, B. (1960) *The Informed Heart.* New York: The Free Press.

Beverage, W. (1942) *Sir William Beverage Announcement.* BBC Radio Home Service Broadcast, 2 December 1942.

Black, D., Blum, N., Pfol, B. and St. John, D. (2004) 'The Stepps Group Treatment Programme for outpatients with borderline personality disorder.' *Journal of Contemporary Psychotherapy 34,* 3, 193–210.

Bloom, S. (1997) *Creating Sanctuary: Towards the Evolution of Sane Societies.* New York: Routledge.

Blum, N., Allen, J., McCormich, B. and Black, D. (2008) 'Letter regarding Randomised Control Trial.' *American Journal of Psychiatry 165,* 10, 1354.

Bond, G.R., Drake, R.E. and Becker, D.R. (2008) 'An update on randomized controlled trials of evidence-based supported employment.' *Psychiatric Rehabilitation Journal 31,* 208–289.

Bowlby, J. (1969) *Attachment and Loss.* London: Hogarth Press.

Bowlby, J. (1988) *A Secure Base.* London: Routledge.

Braun, V. and Clarke, V. (2006) 'Using thematic analysis in psychology.' *Qualitative Research in Psychology 3,* 77–101.

British Psychological Society Division of Clinical Psychology (2000) *Recent Advances in Understanding Mental Illness and Psychotic Experiences.* Leicester: British Psychological Society.

Brower, L.A. (2003) 'The Ohio Mental Health Consumer Outcomes System: Reflections on a Major Policy Initiative in the US.' *Clinical Psychology and Psychotherapy 10,* 400–406.

Burman, E. (1994) 'Feminist Research.' In P. Banister, E. Burman, I. Parker, M. Taylor and C. Tindall (eds.) *Qualitative Methods in Psychology.* Buckingham: Open University Press.

Calnan, J. (2010) *Vital Project's Funding Plea.* Colchester: The Gazette.

Campling, P. and Haigh, R. (1999) *Therapeutic Communities: Past, Present and Future.* London: Jessica Kingsley Publishers.

Campling, P. (1999) 'Chaotic Personalities: Maintaining the Therapeutic Alliance.' In P. Campling and R. Haigh (eds) *Therapeutic Communities: Past, Present and Future.* London: Jessica Kingsley Publishers.

Campling, P. (2001) 'Therapeutic Communities.' *Advances in Psychiatric Treatment 7,* 365–372.

Care Services Improvement Partnership, Royal College of Psychiatrists and Social Care Institute for Excellence (2007) *A Common Purpose: Recovery in Future Mental Health Services.* Leeds: CSIP.

Castillo, H. (2003) *Personality Disorder: Temperament or Trauma?* London: Jessica Kingsley Publishers.

Castillo, H. (2009) 'The Person with a Personality Disorder.' In I. Norman and I. Ryrie (eds) *The Art and Science of Mental Health Nursing,* 2nd edn. Maidenhead: Open University Press.

Castillo, H. (2013) 'Social inclusion and personality disorder.' *Mental Health and Social Inclusion Journal Volume 7,* 3, 147–155.

Castillo, H. and Allen, L. (2003) 'Making Sense of Personality Disorder.' In S. Ramon (ed.) *Users Researching Health and Social Care: An Empowering Agenda?* Birmingham: Ventura.

Castillo, H., Ramon, S. and Morant, N. (2013) 'A recovery journey for people with personality disorder.' *International Journal of Social Psychiatry 59*, 3, 264–273.

Chamberlin, J. (1988) *On our Own*. London: Mind Publications.

Checkland, P. (1999) *Systems Thinking, Systems Practice: Includes a 30-Year Retrospective*. Chichester: Wiley.

Chiesa, M., Bateman, A., Wilberg, T. and Friss, S. (2002) 'Patients' characteristics, outcome and cost-benefit of hospital-based-treatment for patients with a personality disorder: A comparison of three difference programmes.' *Psychology and Psychotherapy: Theory, Research and Practice 75*, 381–392.

Cleckley, H. (1941) *The Mask of Sanity*. St. Louis: CY Mosby Co.

Coid, J., Yang, M., Tyrer, P., Roberts, A. and Ulrich, S. (2006) 'Prevalence and correlates of personality disorder in Great Britain.' *British Journal of Psychiatry 188*, 423–431.

Coleman, R. (1999) *Recovery: An Alien Concept?* Gloucester: Handsell.

Coleman, R. (2014) *DSM Zero – Everything You Need to Know About Your Mental Health*. Isle of Lewis: Working to Recovery.

College of Occupational Therapists (2006) *Recovering Ordinary Lives: The Strategy for Occupational Therapy in Mental Health Services 2007–2017*. London: College of Occupational Therapists.

Cooke, A. and McGowan, J. (2014) *Is Life a Disease? Discursive of Tunbridge Wells*. Canterbury and Christ Church University. Available at http://discursiveoftunbridgewells.blogspot.co.uk/2013/09/is-life-disease.html, accessed on 22 March 2015.

Copeland, M.E. (2001) *The Depression Workbook*. New York: Barnes and Noble.

Crawford, M.J. (2007) *Learning the Lessons: A Multimethod Evaluation of Dedicated Community-Based Services for People with Personality Disorder*. London: HMSO.

Crawford, M.J., Adedeji, T., Price, K. and Rutter, D. (2010) 'Job satisfaction and burnout among staff working in community-based personality disorder services.' *International Journal of Social Psychiatry 56*, 196–206.

Creswell, J.W. (2003) *Research Design, Qualitative, Quantitative, and Mixed Methods Approaches*, 2nd edn. London: Sage.

Davidson, L. (2003) *Living Outside Mental Illness: Qualitative Studies in Schizophrenia*. New York and London: New York University Press.

Daw, R., Spencer-Lane, T., Cobb, A. and Bell, A. (2007) *The Mental Health Act 2007: The Final Report*. The Mental Health Alliance.

Deegan, P. (1988) 'Recovery: the lived experience of rehabilitation.' *Psychosocial Rehabilitation Journal 11*, 11–19.

Deegan, P. (1990) 'How recovery begins.' *The Centre for Community Change Through Housing and Support: VT, CI 25*. Burlington: Trinity College.

Deegan, P. (1993) 'Recovering our sense of value after being labeled mentally ill.' *Journal of Psychosocial Nursing and Mental Health Services 31*, 7–11.

Denman, C. (2001) 'Cognitive-analytic therapy.' *Advances in Psychiatric Treatment 7*, 243–252.

Department of Health (1999) *Managing Dangerous People with Severe Personality Disorder*. London: HMSO.

Department of Health (2003a) *Personality Disorder: No Longer a Diagnosis of Exclusion. Policy Implementation Guidance for the Development of Services for People with Personality Disorder*. London: HMSO.

Department of Health (2003b) *Personality Disorder Capabilities Framework: Breaking the Cycle of Rejection*. London: HMSO.

REFERENCES

Department of Health (2006) *From Values to Action: The Chief Nursing Officer's Review of Mental Health Nursing.* London: HMSO.

Department of Health (2007) *Personality Disorder Knowledge and Understanding Framework.* Available at www.personalitydisorderkuf.org.uk, accessed on 22 March 2015.

Department of Health (2009) *Implementing the NHS Performance Framework: Application to Mental Health Trusts.* London: HMSO.

Department of Health (2014) *Meeting the Challenge, Making a Difference: Working Effectively to Support People with Personality Disorder in the Community.* London: HMSO.

Department of Health and Ministry of Justice (2009) *The Bradley Report.* London: HMSO.

Department of Health and Ministry of Justice (2011) *Response to the Offender Personality Disorder Consultation.* London: HMSO.

Disability Discrimination Act (2005) London: HMSO.

Doering, S., Horz, S., Rentrop, M., Fischer-Kern, M., Schuster, P., Benecke, C., Buchheim, A., Martius, P. and Buchheim, P. (2010) 'Transference-focused psychotherapy v. treatment by community psychotherapists for borderline personality disorder.' *The British Journal of Psychiatry 196*, 389–395.

DSM I (1952) *Diagnostic and Statistical Manual of Mental Disorders,* 1st edn. Washington DC: American Psychiatric Association.

DSM III (1980) *Diagnostic and Statistical Manual of Mental Disorders,* 3st edn. Washington DC: American Psychiatric Association.

DSM IV (1994) *Diagnostic and Statistical Manual of Mental Disorders,* 4th edn. Washington DC: American Psychiatric Association.

DSM 5 (2013) *Diagnostic and Statistical Manual of Mental Disorders,* 5th edn. Washington DC: American Psychiatric Association.

Duggan, C., Adams, C. and McCarthy, L. (2007) *Systematic Review of the Effectiveness of Pharmacological and Psychological Strategies for the Management of People with Personality Disorder.* NHS National R&D Programme in Forensic Mental Health.

Edwards, J. (2012) *Crimes That Shook Britain: The Russell Murders.* The Daily Mirror, 9 May 2012.

Evans, C. and Fisher, F. (1999) 'Collaborative Evaluation with Service Users: Moving Towards User Controlled Research.' In I. Shaw and T. Lishman (eds.) *Evaluation and Social Work Practice.* London: Sage.

Faulkner, A., Petit-Zeman, S., Sherlock, J. and Wallcraft, J. (2002) *Being There in a Crisis.* London: Mental Health Foundation and Sainsbury Centre for Mental Health.

Feigenbaum, J. (2007) 'Dialectical behaviour therapy: An increasing evidence base.' *Journal of Mental Health 16,* 1, 51–68.

Fonagy, P. (1997) *When Cure is Inconceivable: The Aims of Psychoanalysis with Borderline Patients.* Paper to New York Freudian Society, 4 April 1997.

Fonagy, P. and Bateman, A. (2008) 'The development of borderline personality disorder: a mentalizing model.' *Journal of Personality Disorders 22,* 1, 4–21.

Freire, P. (1970) *Pedagogy of the Oppressed.* New York: Herder and Herder.

French, G.D. and Harris C.J. (1998) *Traumatic Incident Reduction.* London and New York: Taylor and Francis.

Fuller, B. (2002) *Critical Path.* New York: Saint Martin's Griffin.

Fuller, R. and Petch, A. (1995) *Practitioner Research.* Buckingham: Open University Press.

Gans, S. and Grohol, J.M. (2010) 'Transference-focused therapy, Dialectical behaviour therapy, Schema Therapy and Mentalization-based therapy.' Adapted from articles by The American

Psychiatric Association. Available at www.bpdresources.net/top_articles/bpd_therapy.htm, accessed on 22 March 2014.

Goffman, E. (1963) *Stigma: Notes on the Management of Spoiled Identity*. London: Penguin.

Gorman, H. (1999) 'Practitioner Research in Community Care: Personalising the Political.' In B. Broad (ed.) *The Politics of Social Work Research and Evaluation*. Birmingham: Ventura Press.

Gostin, L.O. (1975) *A Human Condition: Volume I*. London: Mind Publications.

Gregory, R.J. (2004) 'Thematic stages of recovery in the treatment of borderline personality disorder.' *American Journal of Psychotherapy 58*, 3, 335–348.

Gutheil, T. and Gabbard, G.O. (1993) 'The Concept of Boundaries in Clinical Practice; Theoretical and Risk-management Dimensions.' In G. Adshed and C. Jacob (eds.) *Personality Disorder: The Definitive Reader*. London: Jessica Kingsley Publishers.

Haigh, R. (1999) 'The Quintessence of a Therapeutic Environment: Five Universal Qualities.' In P. Campling and R. Haigh (eds.) *Therapeutic Communities: Past, Present and Future*. London: Jessica Kingsley Publishers.

Haigh, R. (2003) 'Services for People with Personality Disorder: The Thoughts of Service Users.' In *Personality Disorder: No Longer a Diagnosis of Exclusion*. Policy Implementation Guidance for the Development of Services for People with Personality Disorder. London: HMSO.

Hammersley, M. (1989) *The Dilemma of Qualitative Method: Herbert Bulmer and the Chicago Tradition*. London: Routledge.

Harding, C.M., Brooks, G.W., Asologa, Y.S.J.S. and Brier, A. (1987) 'The Vermont longitudinal studies of persons with severe mental illness.' *American Journal of Psychiatry 144*, 718–726.

Harvey, R. (2009) *Stepps Programme*. Presentation to Haven Staff, 8 July 2009.

Health and Social Care Act (2012) London: HMSO.

Henderson, D. (1939) *Psychopathic States*. New York: W.E. Norton.

Henwood, K.L. and Pidgeon, N.F. (1994) 'Qualitative Research and Psychological Theorising.' In M. Hammersley (ed.) *Social Research: Philosophy, Politics and Practice*. London: Sage.

Herman, J. and Van der Kolk, B. (1987) *Traumatic Origins of Borderline Personality Disorder in Psychological Trauma*. Washington DC: American Psychiatric Press.

Hinshelwood, R.D. (1996) 'Communities and their health.' *Therapeutic Communities 17*, 173–182.

Hinshelwood, R.D. (1998) 'The difficult patient: The role of "scientific psychiatry" in understanding patients with chronic schizophrenia or severe personality disorder.' *British Journal of Psychotherapy 174*, 187–190.

Hinshelwood, R.D. (1999) 'Psychoanalytic Origins and Today's Work; The Cassel Heritage.' In P. Campling and R. Haigh (eds.) *Therapeutic Communities: Past, Present and Future*. London: Jessica Kingsley Publishers.

HMSO (2009a) *New Horizons: A Shared Vision for Mental Health*. London: HMSO.

HMSO (2009b) *Work Recovery and Inclusion: Employment support for people in contact with secondary mental health services*. London: HMSO.

Hogan, M.F. (2001) *Vital Signs: A Statewide Approach to Measuring Consumer Outcomes in Ohio's Publicly-Supported Community Mental Health System*. Final Report of the Ohio Mental Health Outcomes Task Force.

Howard, L.M., Heslin, M., Leese, M., McCrone, P., Rice, C., Jarrett, M., Spokes, T., Huxley, P. and Thornicroft, G. (2010) 'Supported employment: randomized controlled trial.' *British Journal of Psychiatry 196*, 404–411.

ICD 10 (1992) *Classification of Mental and Behavioural Disorders*. Geneva: World Health Organization.

Jung, C.G. (1954) *The Psychology of the Transference from The Collected Works of C.G. Jung*. New York: Bollingen Foundation.

Kabat-Zinn, J. (2001) *Full Catastrophe Living: Using the Wisdom of your Body and Mind to Face Stress and Illness*. London: Piatkus Books.

Katasakou, C., Marougka, S., Barnicot, K., Savill, M., White, H., Lockwood, K. and Priebe, S. (2012) 'Recovery in Borderline Personality Disorder (BPD): A qualitative study of service users' perspectives.' *PloS ONE 7*, 5.

Kernberg, O. (1984) *Severe Personality Disorders: Psychotherapeutic Strategies*. London: Yale University Press.

Kerr, I.B. (2001) *The Difficult Patient*. Presentation at South London and Maudsley Mental Health NHS Trust Conference on Personality Disorder on 9 May 2001.

Kerr, I.B. (2006) 'Cognitive-analytic therapy for borderline personality disorder in the context of a community mental health team: Individual and organisational psychodynamic implications.' *British Journal of Psychotherapy 5*, 4, 425–438.

Koch, J.L.A. (1891) *Die Psychopathischen Minderwertigkeiten*. Ravensburg, Germany: Maier.

Kofman, F. and Senge, P. (2001) *Communities of Commitment; The Heart of Learning Organisations*. Organisational Learning Centre, Cambridge USA: Massachusetts Institute of Technology.

Kolakowski, L. (1995) 'An Overall View of Positivism.' In P. Reason (ed.) *Human Inquiry in Action*. London: Sage.

Kraepelin, E. (1905) 'Personality Disorder' In M. Gelder, D. Gath and R. Mayou (eds.) *Oxford Text Book of Psychiatry*, 2nd edn. Published in 1989. Oxford: Oxford Medical Publications.

Lawton-Smith, S. (2012) *Employment is vital for maintaining good mental health*. London: Mental Health Foundation.

Lees, J., Manning, N. and Rawlings, B. (1999) *Therapeutic Community Effectiveness. A Systematic International Review of Therapeutic Community Treatment for People with Personality Disorders and Mentally Disordered Offenders:* CRD Report 17: York: NHS Centre for Reviews and Dissemination.

Leete, E. (1989) 'How I perceive and manage my illness.' *Schizophrenia Bulletin 15*, 197–200.

Lewis, G. and Appleby, L. (1988) 'Personality disorder: The patients psychiatrists dislike.' *British Journal of Psychiatry 153*, 44–49.

Liberman, R.P. and Kopelowicz, A. (2005) 'Recovery from schizophrenia: A concept in search of research.' *Psychiatric Services: ps.psychiatryonline.org 56*, 6, 735–742.

Linehan, M.M. (1993) *Skills Training Manual for Treating Borderline Personality Disorder*. New York and London: Guilford Press.

Linehan, M.M. (2011) *The Power of Rescuing Others*. The New York Times, 23 June 2011, p. A1.

Linehan, M.M., Armstrong, H.E., Suarez, A., Allmon, D. and Heard, H.L. (1991) 'Cognitive-behavioural treatment of chronically parasuicidal borderline patients.' *Archives of General Psychiatry 50*, 971–974.

Lombroso, C. (1876) 'Illustrative Studies in Criminal Anthropology.' *Monist 1*, 177–176.

Lucas, C. (2014) *We Need a More Courageous, Robust Response If We're to Save Our NHS*. Huff Post Politics, 21 November 2014.

Mahari, A.J. (2004) *BPD from the inside out: Why Boundaries?* Available at www.borderlinepersonality. ca.borderlinewhyboundaries.htm, accessed on 22 March 2015.

Main, T.F. (1967) 'Knowledge, learning and freedom from thought.' *Australia and New Zealand Journal of Psychiatry 1,* 64–67. Re-printed in 1990 in *Psychoanalytic Psychotherapy 5,* 49–78.

Marshall, M.N. (1996) 'Sampling for Qualitative Research.' *Family Practice 13.* Oxford University Press.

Maslow, A.H. (1943) 'A theory of human motivation.' *Psychological Review 50,* 4, 370–396.

Maudsley, H. (1884) In Kutchins, H. and Kirk, S.A. (eds.) Published in 1999. *Making us Crazy: DSM The Psychiatric Bible and the Creation of Mental Disorders.* London: Constable.

McCrone, P., Dhanasiri, S., Patel, A., Knapp, S. and Lawton-Smith, S. (2008) *Playing the Price: The Cost of Mental Health Care in England to 2026.* London: The Kings Fund.

McGowan, J. (2009) 'Use your loaf: Open up choice.' *Health Service Journal 2 July 2009,* 15.

McGowan, J. (2010) 'It's time we shattered a great NHS myth and said that service-user involvement is often of little or no use.' *Health Service Journal 27 May 2010,* 14–15.

Mental Deficiency Act (1913) London: HMSO.

Mental Health Act (1959) London: HMSO.

Mental Health Act (1983) London: HMSO.

Mental Health Act (2007) London: HMSO.

Menzies, D., Dolan, B. and Norton, K. (1993) 'Funding treatment for personality disorders: are short term savings worth long term costs?' *Psychiatric Bulletin 7,* 517–519.

Monbiot, G. (2014) *Taming corporate power: the key political issue of our age.* The Guardian, 8 December 2014.

Moran, P. (2007) 'Psychotherapy for BPD gets growing evidence base.' *Psychiatric News 42,* 2, 26. American Psychiatric Association.

Morel, B.A. (1857) *Treatise on the Intellectual, Moral, and Physical Degeneracy of the Human Race.* Paris: Baillière.

National Health Service Act (1946) London: HMSO.

National Health Service and Community Care Act (1990) London: HMSO.

National Health Service Reform and Health Care Professions Act (2002) London: HMSO.

National Health Service (Amended Duties and Powers) Bill (2014) Available at www.parliament. uk/business/publications/research/briefing-papers/SN07026/national-health-service-amended-duties-and-powers-bill-bill-18-of-201415, accessed on 22 March 2015.

Nehls, N. (2000) 'Recovering: A process of empowerment.' *Advanced Nursing Science 22,* 4, 62–70.

Nevis, E.C., DiBella, A.J. and Gould, J.M. (1995) 'Understanding organisations as learning systems.' *MIT Sloan Management Review: Winter 1995,* p.3626.

NICE (2009) *Borderline Personality Disorder: treatment and management.* NICE Clinical Guideline 78. National Institute for Health and Clinical Excellence. NHS.

NICE (2010) *Antisocial Personality Disorder: treatment and management.* NICE Clinical Guideline 77. National Institute for Health and Clinical Excellence. NHS.

NIMHE (2005) *NIMHE Guiding Statement on Mental Health Recovery.* London: National Institute for Mental Health England.

Norton, K. and Bloom, S.L. (2004) 'The art and challenges of long-term and short-term democratic therapeutic communities.' *Psychiatric Quarterly 75,* 3, 249–261.

O'Connar, J. (2001) *NLP Workbook.* London and New York: Harper Collins.

Onken, S.J. (2004) *User Perspectives on Mental Health Recovery Facilitating and Hindering Factors.* The Fourth International Conference on Social Work in Health and Mental Health, Quebec City, Canada, May 23–27.

Padilla, R.V. (1993) 'Using Dialogical Research Methods in Group Interviews.' In D.L. Morgan (ed.) *Successful Focus Groups: Advancing the State of the Art.* London: Sage.

Paris, J. (2004) 'Half in love with easeful death: The meaning of chronic suicidality in borderline personality disorder.' *Harvard Review of Psychiatry 12,* 42–48.

Parker, I. (1994) 'Qualitative Research.' In P. Banister, E. Burman, I. Parker, M. Taylor and C. Tindall (eds.). *Qualitative Methods in Psychology.* Buckingham: Open University Press.

Percival, W. (1961) *A Patient's Account of his Psychosis.* Stanford, California: Stanford University Press.

Perkins, R. (1999) 'The individual's journey: Recovery and service provision.' *Psychological News 2,* 1. Bromley Psychosocial Rehabilitation Forum.

Perkins, R., Farmer, P. and Litchfield, P. (2009) *Realising Ambitions: Better Employment Support for People with a Mental Health Condition.* November 2009. London: Department of Work and Pensions.

Perry, J.C., Banon, E. and Ianni, F. (1999) 'Effectiveness of psychotherapy for personality disorders.' *American Journal of Psychiatry 156,* 1312–1321.

Pilgrim, D. (2000) *Construct Validity in Personality Trait Theory.* Seminar presented in relation to the results of dissertation by H. Castillo, *Personality Disorder, Temperament or Trauma?* Chelmsford: Anglia Polytechnic University.

Pinel, P. (1801) In M. Gelder, D. Gath and R. Mayou (eds.) 'Personality Disorder' (Ref. Kauka,1949, for translation) In *Oxford Text Book of Psychiatry,* 2nd edn. Published in 1989. Oxford: Oxford Medical Publications.

Pollock, A. (2014) *Privatisation of the NHS.* A TEDxExeter talk. Available at www.youtube.com/watch?v=Cz5dl9fhj7o, accessed on 22 March 2015.

Porter, M. (2014) *Health Boss Claims Personality Disorder Service Does not Reach Enough People.* Colchester Daily Gazette, 29 October 2014.

Pritchard, J.C. (1835) In M. Gelder, D. Gath and R. Mayou (eds.) 'Personality Disorder'. In *Oxford Text Book of Psychiatry,* 2nd edn. Published in 1989. Oxford: Oxford Medical Publications.

Ramesh, R. (2011*) Labour's fight against NHS competition is 'depressing', Alan Milburn complains.* The Guardian, 12 December 2011.

Ramon, S. (2011) 'Organizational change in the context of recovery oriented services.' *Journal of Mental Health Training, Education and Practice: Issue for Workforce Development 6,* 1, 37–45.

Ramon, S., Castillo, H. and Morant, N. (2001) 'Experiencing personality disorder.' *International Journal of Social Psychiatry 47,* 4, 1–15.

Ramon, S., Healey, B. and Renouf, N. (2007) 'Recovery from mental illness as an emergent concept and practice in Australia and the UK.' *International Journal of Social Psychiatry 53,* 2, 108–122.

Rapoport, R.N. (1960) *Community as Doctor.* London: Tavistock.

Rawlinson, D. (1999) 'Group Analytic Ideas; Extending the Group Matrix into TCs.' In P. Campling and R. Haigh (eds.) *Therapeutic Communities: Past, Present and Future.* London: Jessica Kingsley Publishers.

Reeves, A. (1999) *Recovery: A Holistic Approach.* Gloucester: Handsell Publishing.

Repper, J. and Perkins, R. (2003) *Social Inclusion and Recovery: A Model for Mental Health Practice.* London and New York: Bailliere Tindall.

Rey, J.H. (1994) *Universals of Psychoanalysis in the Treatment of Psychotic and Borderline States.* London: Free Association Books.

Roberts, G. and Wolfson, P. (2004) 'The rediscovery of recovery: open to all.' *Advances in Psychiatric Treatment, 10,* 37–49.

Roberts, G. and Wolfson, P. (2006) 'New directions in rehabilitation: learning from the recovery movement' In G. Roberts, S. Davenport, F. Holloway and T. Tattan (eds.) *Enabling Recovery: The Principles and Practice of Rehabilitation Psychiatry.* London: Gaskell.

Robson, C. (1997) *Real World Research: A Resource for Social Scientists and Practitioner Researchers.* Oxford: Blackwell.

Roderick, P. and Pollock, A. (2014) *The Proposed NHS Reinstatement Bill.* Centre for Primary Care and Public Health, University of London.

Rollnick, S., Miller, W.R. and Butler, C.C. (1995) *Motivational Interviewing in Healthcare.* New York and London: Guilford Press.

Roth, M.A., Crane-Ross, D., Hannon, M.J. and Cusick, G.M. (2000) 'A Longitudinal Study of Mental Health Services and Consumer Outcomes in a Changing System: Time 5 Results.' *New Research in Mental Health, 14,* 159–176. Columbus, OH: The Ohio Department of Mental Health.

Rowan, J. and Reason, P. (1981) *Human Inquiry a Source Book of New Paradigm Research.* Chichester: Wiley.

Russinova, Z. (1999) 'Providers' hope-inspiring competence as a factor optimising psychiatric rehabilitation outcomes.' *Journal of Rehabilitation Oct–Dec,* 50–57.

Ryle, A. (1997) *Cognitive Analytic Therapy: The Model and the Method.* Chichester: Wiley.

Schneider, K. (1923) *Psychopathic Personalities.* London: Cassell.

Senge, P.M. (1990) *The Fifth Discipline: The Art and Practice of the Learning Organisation.* New York: Doubleday.

Shepherd, A., Doyle, M., Sanders, C and Shaw, J. (2015) 'Personal recovery within forensic settings – Systematic review and meta-synthesis of qualitative methods studies'. *Criminal Behaviour and Mental Health.* Wiley Online Library (wileyonlinelibrary.com) DOI: 10.1002/cbm.1966.

Slade, M., Amering, M. and Oades, L. (2008) 'Recovery: An international perspective.' *Epidemiolofia e Psychatria Sociale 17,* 2, 128–137.

Smith, J.A. (2003) *Qualitative Psychology.* London: Sage.

Social Exclusion Task Force (2006) *Reaching Out: An Action Plan on Social Exclusion.* London. HM Cabinet Office.

Stalker, K., Ferguson, I. and Barclay, A. (2005) 'It is a horrible term for someone'. Service user and provider perspectives on personality disorder.' *Disability and Society 20,* 4, 359–373.

Stanton, A. (1989) *Invitation to Self-Management.* Ruislip: Dab Hand Press.

Szasz, T.S. (1961) *The Myth of Mental Illness.* London: Secker and Warburg.

Tait, L., Birchwood, M. and Trower, P. (2003) 'Predicting engagement with services for psychosis: insight, symptoms and recovery style.' *British Journal of Psychiatry 182,* 123–128.

Thorlby, R. and Maybin J. (eds.) (2010) *A high-performing NHS? A Review of the Evidence 1997–2010.* London: The King's Fund.

Tindall, C. (1994) *Qualitative Methods in Psychology.* Buckingham: Open University Press.

Tolkien, J.R.R. (1954) *The Fellowship of the Ring.* New York: Houghton Mifflin.

Tomlinson, D. and Carrier, J. (1996) *Asylum in the Community.* London and New York: Routledge.

Topor, A. (2004) *What Helps People Recover?* Keynote Speech to the Annual NIMHE Eastern Conference, 23 September 2004.

REFERENCES

Tucker, S. (1999) 'The Therapeutic Approach and Learning to Care.' In P. Campling and R. Haigh (eds.) *Therapeutic Communities: Past, Present and Future.* London: Jessica Kingsley Publishers.

Turner-Crowson, J. and Wallcraft, J. (2002) 'The recovery vision for mental health services and research: A British perspective.' *Psychiatric Rehabilitation Journal 25,* 3, 245–254.

Turner, K., Lovell, K. and Brooker, A. (2011) '… And they all lived happily ever after: "recovery" or discovery of the self in personality disorder?' *Psychodynamic Practice 17,* p.3.

Tyrer, P. (1988) *Personality Disorder, Management and Care.* London: Wright.

Unzicker, R. (1989) 'On my own: A personal journey through madness and re-emergence.' *Psychosocial Rehabilitation Journal 13,* 1, 71–77.

Van der Kolk, B. (1989) 'The compulsion to repeat trauma: Re-enactment, re-victimization and masochism.' *Psychiatric Clinics of North America 12,* 389–411.

Van der Kolk, B. (1996) *Traumatic Stress.* London and New York: Guilford Press.

Wallcraft, J. (2005) 'The Place of Recovery.' In S. Ramon and J. Williams (eds.) *Mental Health at the Crossroads: The Promise of the Psychological Approach.* Abingdon: Ashgate.

Wallcraft, J. (2011) 'Service users' perceptions of quality of life measurement in psychiatry.' *Advances in Psychiatric Treatment 17,* 266–274.

Warren, F. and Dolan B. (2001) *Perspectives on Henderson Hospital.* Sutton: Henderson Hospital.

Whittaker, A. (2009) *Research Skills for Social Work.* Exeter: Learning Matters.

Winnicott, D. (1965) *The Maturational Process and the Facilitating Environment.* London: Hogarth.

Winnicott, D. (1971) *Playing and Reality.* London: Tavistock.

Winter, R. and Munn-Giddings, C. (2001) *A Handbook for Action Research in Health and Social Care.* London: Routledge.

Wrench, M. (2012) 'Annihilating the Other: Forensic Aspects of Organisational Change.' In J. Adlam, A. Aiyegbusi, P. Kleinot, A. Motz and C. Scanlon (eds.) *The Therapeutic Milieu Under Fire.* London: Jessica Kingsley Publishers.

Wynne-Jones, R. (2015) *The lifesaving clinic being closed by government cuts.* The Mirror, 27 January 2015.

Yeomans, F.E., Clarkin, J.F. and Kernberg, O.F. (2002) *A Primer of Transference-Focused Psychotherapy for the Borderline Patient.* Lanham, MD: Rowman and Littlefield.

Young, J.E., Klosko, J.S. and Weishaar, M.E. (2003) *Schema Therapy A Practitioner's Guide.* New York and London: Guilford Press.

Zanarini, M.C., Frankenburg, F.R., Reich, D.B. and Fitzmaurice, G. (2012) 'Attainment and stability of sustained symptomatic remission and recovery among patients with borderline personality disorder and axis II comparison subjects: A 16-year prospective follow-up study.' *American Journal Psychiatry 169,* 476–483.

Zeller, R.A. (1993) 'Focus Group Research on Sensitive Topics.' In D.L. Morgan (ed.) *Successful Focus Groups: Advancing the State of the Art.* London: Sage.

Subject Index

Page numbers in *italics* refer to figures and tables.

Author Index